Hypnotherapy: everything you need to know about hypnosis and how it can help you

HYPNOTHERAPY:

everything you need to know
about hypnosis and how
it can help you

Dr. Ruth Lever Kidson

Sussex: Sphinx House Publishing

Published by Sphinx House Publishing
East Sussex BN2 8FL

ABOUT THE AUTHOR

Dr. Ruth Lever Kidson is a qualified physician, medical
hypnotherapist and psychotherapist.

Other books by Ruth Lever Kidson:

Insomnia and Other Sleep Disorders
Is Acupuncture Right for You?
A Guide to Common Illnesses

CONTENTS

CHAPTER ONE: WHAT IS HYPNOSIS?

Hypnosis has had a bad press for many years and it's still its seedier aspects with which many people are familiar. The word itself, rather than conjuring up the idea of a safe and simple therapy, used by many doctors and dentists worldwide to treat a wide range of ailments, may just as easily make them think of a gold watch swinging on a long chain and the words "You are falling asleep . . . you cannot resist . . ." being muttered in a foreign accent. Or they may think of people being made to behave like three year olds, unaware that everyone else is laughing at them. Those who have come across Gillian Cross's series of children's books about *The Demon Headmaster* may even remember how the Headmaster uses hypnosis to control everyone who gets in his way, in his bid to take over the world.

This image problem really started with Dr. Franz Anton Mesmer, the father of hypnosis, who, with his extroverted and somewhat outlandish ways (which will be described in chapter two) alienated many of his fellow doctors, despite the fact that he was a successful practitioner. And, of course, in more recent times, thriller writers and film makers have been unable to resist the concept of a simple technique which appears to give its user the power to control other people.

Admittedly, in the past few decades, people have become more aware that hypnosis can be used as a therapy, if only because many have tried it to help them give up smoking. And here again, of course, the impression is of people being made to do things against their will—heavy smokers being *made* to give up their cigarettes.

So it's understandable that, even in those cases where people have been advised by their doctors to consult a hypnotherapist, they may do so with considerable trepidation, not knowing quite what hypnotherapists do — or, perhaps more importantly, don't do.

What they *don't* do is control their patients' minds. Which is just as well because, if this really were the case, who knows what might happen if you were unfortunate enough to get into the hands of an unscrupulous practitioner. I'm reminded of some lines from a classic comedy show I heard on the radio. One of the characters is hypnotizing another and says "Now open your purse and repeat after me . . . Help yourself." If hypnosis really did work in this way, it would be possible for the subjects to be made to do all sorts of things against their will — even commit crimes or divulge secrets that they would rather keep hidden, making it very like brainwashing. Fortunately, it's not like this at all (and if it were, I suspect that it would have been made illegal long ago) and hypnosis can't make you do anything to which you would normally object.

For all those people who have been helped to give up smoking with hypnosis, there are others who have carried on smoking despite the treatment — clear proof that a hypnotherapist can't make you do anything you don't want to. Invariably, you will find that those who did give up were strongly motivated, so that the hypnosis was able to reinforce their own determination to quit, strengthening their will-power and making the transition from smoker to nonsmoker a lot easier than it might otherwise have been. When hypnosis fails, it tends to be with people who don't really want to give up, for whom smoking is a pleasure rather than just a habit. They try hypnosis because they feel that they ought to give up—perhaps pressure is being put on them by partners, parents or doctors—or they may have financial or health reasons for wanting to stop. But whatever the reason, it's not strong enough. The desire isn't there, and hypnosis can't create something out of nothing.

Of course, the question then arises—if hypnotists aren't truly in control of their subjects' minds, how come stage hypnotists can get people to do daft things? The answer is, in fact, quite simple, although you need to look at the whole of the hypnotist's act in order to understand how it works. He (it's almost always a man) will usually start by asking everyone in the audience to do a few tests, so he can see who is likely to be a good hypnotic subject. The tests are introduced as a sort of game, so the audience doesn't realize it's being tested and, by the time the 'game' is over, everyone will be in a party mood and ready to join in the show.

Then the hypnotist will pick out a number of people who, from the way they responded to the tests, seem as though they're likely to be good subjects, and he'll ask them to come up on stage. Anyone who doesn't want to join in is likely to refuse at this point. So you can be fairly sure that all those who actually climb up onto the stage are willing subjects and, as long as they're not asked to do something completely against their principles (such as taking their clothes off) they'll play along with the act. Next, the hypnotist will do some more tests with the people on stage and, out of the 15 or 20 he initially picked out, he'll choose perhaps five or six who seem to him to be both good subjects and good sports.

A few years before I became interested in hypnotherapy, I was at a nightclub where part of the cabaret was a hypnotism act. I was one of those invited to 'come up on stage' and I was chosen as one of the final four subjects. We were asked to do various silly things which I knew perfectly well were silly at the time—but I went along with them because it was a bit of fun and I didn't want to spoil the man's act. That's not to say, however, that hypnosis is always safe—I'll go into the dangers of stage hypnosis in chapter four. And it's always possible for subjects to become upset or embarrassed when they find themselves doing silly things. But any suggestion which the subject finds truly objectionable will be ignored.

However, hypnotism as used by stage hypnotists really has very little in common with hypnotherapy other than the basic technique. It's important to remember that the sole aim of the stage hypnotist is to entertain and, in order to do that, he may make hypnosis look quite different from what it actually is. His subjects, as we have seen, are willing to 'join in the fun' and so are unlikely to resist hypnosis. But it's perfectly possible to refuse to go into a trance—indeed it's impossible to hypnotize anyone who is unwilling to be hypnotized. (Paradoxically, it's also very hard to get people to go into a trance if they're too keen to do so. It's like willing yourself to go to sleep—it just doesn't work.)

However, patients who have been reassured about what can and can't be done with hypnosis are usually fairly relaxed about the induction and go under quite easily. And the more often you're hypnotized, the easier it gets, because you become more confident both about the technique itself and about its benefits. But it is vital that, from the word go, the patient knows that it is he (or she) who is in control and not the therapist. (From now on, unless I'm talking specifically about a female patient or therapist, I'm going to use 'he' rather than 'he or she'. I know there are female therapists—I'm one myself and I know there are female patients—I've been one of those, too! I'm sorry if this offends anyone but I find the constant repetition of 'he or she' very irritating and, having been taught English grammar by a teacher 'of the old school', I object strongly to using 'they' to refer to a single individual.)

So—the patient is in control. That needs to be made clear from the start. Because he is control, he can't be made to stay in hypnosis if he decides that he wants to wake up. Usually patients enjoy being in a trance and have no wish to cut the session short, but occasionally someone will bring himself out, and it's not uncommon, after the first session, for a patient to say "I felt that I could wake up at any time." (If you ask why he didn't, the answer is usually "Oh, I didn't *want* to—I just felt that I *could*."). However, occasionally the patient may want to wake. He may wake automatically if a suggestion is made that is so contrary to his own ideas that he finds it offensive or alarming—an additional safeguard against being made to do anything against your will. But there may be other reasons. I remember one afternoon when my clinic was running about 20 minutes late and suddenly, half way through her session, my patient woke up and said "I'm terribly sorry, but I've got to go and pick the children up from school." So even though she was in a moderately deep

5

trance, she was aware of the time and of what she had to do and was able to wake herself up in order to do it.

We always tend to talk about waking up from hypnosis and about hypnotic sleep, so it's inevitable that people who've never been hypnotized should imagine that there's little difference between being in a trance and being asleep. And anyone who speaks Greek will know that the word 'hypnosis'is derived from the Greek word for sleep, *hypnos*. So the very word itself can make patients apprehensive — having things 'done to you' while you're asleep is reminiscent of having an operation — something that, understandably, most people are quite nervous about. But the word is misleading. A person asleep is often described as 'dead to the world' but the hypnotized patient is far from being oblivious to everything going on around him and, on the contrary, is able to hear and respond to everything that the therapist says.

However, this is not to say that the patient in hypnosis will respond to his environment in exactly the same way as if he were unhypnotized. Imagine a man and his wife visiting a hypnotherapist together. If the man sits with his eyes closed while his wife and the therapist talk, he may well, at some point, open his eyes and join in the conversation — it just depends on how interested he is in the topic being discussed.

Now imagine that he has already been put into a light trance. In this case, he will listen to the conversation going on but, even if the subject interests him, he'll feel no great desire to join in. If he has gone into a fairly deep trance, however, although he'll continue to hear and understand what is being said, he won't actively listen. But it must be stressed that at no time is the patient 'unconscious', whatever the depth of the trance. Patients who have been regressed under hypnosis (I cover regression in chapter five) may have the most vivid experiences of past events or even what seem to be past lives, but even in the midst of these experiences, they are conscious of where they really are and they will hear the hypnotherapist when he speaks to them.

Under hypnosis, patients are still aware of their surroundings but they become distanced from them. This was nicely demonstrated to me soon after I started my practice as a hypnotherapist. I had put a patient into a trance and was just beginning to give her some suggestions regarding her problem when the 'phone on my desk started to ring. It was quickly answered on the extension but I was concerned that it might have disturbed her. At the end of the session, after I'd woken her up, I asked her about this and she said "Oh, no, it didn't disturb me at all—but I was aware that it had disturbed you!"

Hypnosis is not a form of unconsciousness but, rather, an altered state of consciousness. And the reason it's so useful in therapy is that, in this altered state, a corridor is opened between the conscious and the subconscious mind and the patient becomes more responsive to suggestion than he would normally be. Both our automatic reactions and our response to stress are products of the subconscious mind. Migraine, rashes, asthma and a host of other problems can be brought on by stress. The subconscious also bottles up memories of things that have happened in the past—things that, on the surface, have been forgotten—and sometimes this can result in the development of phobias or abnormal reactions to certain situations. If one can speak to the subconscious mind in the hypnotic state, it may be able to recognize that certain memories are no longer relevant and this may enable it to accept suggestions that it can use to promote beneficial, rather than harmful, automatic reactions.

Let's suppose that someone who wants to give up smoking has gone to see a hypnotherapist. Once he's in a trance, he'll be given certain suggestions to help him quit—perhaps he'll be told that cigarettes will taste dreadful in future and that he'll have no desire to smoke. Now, if he was fully awake, he'd be saying to himself "But I like the taste—and if it was that easy, I'd have given up ages ago." And if he was asleep—or in a state resembling sleep—he wouldn't hear the therapist, so all the suggestions would be lost on him. But in hypnosis, although he is fully aware of what the therapist is saying, the trance has the effect of temporarily removing the brain's critical faculty—in other words, the mind accepts the suggestion that this will happen, without wondering why on earth it should. So the patient will believe what he's been told about evil-tasting cigarettes and his lack of desire to smoke.

Oddly enough, even if the hypnotized patient feels uncertain about the validity of the suggestion, it may still work. I had a patient who came to see me because, as soon as she got upset about anything, she tended to develop a migraine. Unfortunately, she was going through a period when she had a lot of problems and she was getting upset frequently. The resulting increase in the frequency of her migraines was adding to her distress and she found herself in a highly unpleasant vicious cycle. She wasn't convinced that hypnotherapy would help her but she was getting desperate and was prepared to try anything.

Once in hypnosis, she was told that she would be able to cope with her problems, that she'd be able to remain calm and detached, not allowing things to upset her, and that, consequently, she'd stop developing migraines. After I'd woken her up, however, she confessed that, while I'd been saying all these reassuring things, her conscious mind had been retorting "That's what you think!" In view of this, her chances of getting better seemed small. But, to my surprise (and no doubt to hers), when she came for her next appointment, she reported that not only was she coping better and staying calmer but the frequency of her migraines had decreased dramatically.

Although this patient was able to 'answer back' with her conscious mind, her subconscious mind had obviously accepted the suggestions that I'd given her, because they were in her best interests. This is the important thing — the subconscious mind has got to believe that following the suggestions will be beneficial.

When I first became interested in hypnotherapy I attended a series of training courses run by the British Society of Medical and Dental Hypnosis. At one point, one of the tutors wanted to demonstrate that it's possible to make a patient forget certain things while in hypnosis. Choosing me as the subject, he hypnotized me and then told me that when he tapped his pen on the table, I would forget my name for 30 seconds. But I didn't want to forget my name—even for 30 seconds. The very idea made me feel insecure and I wasn't going to do it. And my subconscious mind evidently knew that there was no reason to override this conscious decision. So, when the tutor tapped the table with his pen and then asked me what my name was, I told him. "Ah," he said, "she obviously doesn't want to forget her name. Let's try something less threatening." So he told me that when he tapped the table the next time, I'd forget where I lived. But I didn't want to forget that either, so the same thing happened—he tapped his pen on the table and asked me my address, and I told him.

It will be clear from these various anecdotes that it's quite normal for a subject to remember everything that has happened while he was in a trance. The idea that you forget everything that has occurred as soon as you wake is yet another popular myth—and quite an alarming one, giving hypnosis similar properties to date-rape drugs. But this is fiction. It is, however, the stuff that novels are made of—the hero is hypnotized and only you, the reader, know what instructions he has been given, since he awakes unable to remember anything that has been said. But in fact, it's quite rare for patients spontaneously to forget what has happened while they were in hypnosis. Those that do will have been in a very deep trance, and such deep levels are uncommon. For a start, not all subjects are capable of going very deep. And, of those that can, only a few will be able to do so without considerable work on the part of the hypnotist. For most types of treatment, a very deep trance is unnecessary, so it tends only to occur in the very few who are naturally deep subjects. The vast majority of patients will go into a light or medium depth trance, from which they will emerge remembering everything.

Occasionally, though, there may be reasons why the patient needs to forget something that has come up while he is under hypnosis. For example, he may have developed a phobia as the result of a frightening incident that happened when he was a child. Although the incident was blotted from his conscious mind, the fear that was associated with it remained and has turned into a phobia. In order to treat the condition, it may be important to resurrect the memory of that event while he is in hypnosis, but it may still be too much for his conscious mind to deal with. So, before bringing the patient out of the trance, the therapist may say something along the lines of "You will forget anything that has emerged during this session that your conscious mind is not yet ready to deal with. When—and only when—your conscious mind can cope with them, these memories will slowly come back to you." So it's the patient's own subconscious mind that determines what he remembers, and when. However, as I demonstrated when I refused to forget my name and address, the act of forgetting has got to have some benefit to the subject in order for the subconscious mind to accept it.

The title of this chapter is 'What is Hypnosis' but from what I've said so far, you can see that it's a lot easier to describe hypnosis in terms of what it isn't than in terms of what it is. This may, of course, be the reason why it has never been given a name that really describes what it is or does. 'Hypnosis' is misleading because it implies sleep. Previous names are equally vague. In the seventeenth and eighteenth centuries it was known as 'animal magnetism' in the mistaken belief that it had something to do with the flow of magnetic forces through the subject (more on this in the next chapter). In the following century the magnetic theory became discredited and the term 'animal magnetism' was replaced by 'mesmerism', after Dr. Franz Anton Mesmer, who is seen as the father of modern hypnotherapy. This term is still used, particularly in the sense of "I was mesmerized by it", meaning "I was enthralled". It was only in the mid-nineteenth century that the term 'hypnosis' was coined—the latest in a series of names for a very ancient technique.

CHAPTER TWO: A SHORT HISTORY OF HYPNOSIS

Hypnosis is not a recent discovery. It seems likely that induced hypnotic trances were used therapeutically in the ancient Indian, Greek and Egyptian civilisations, although the people who used them probably regarded them as a form of sleep. But, by the eleventh century, the Persian physician Avicenna, writing about this 'pleasant dreamy state' in his *Book of Healing*, recognized that hypnosis was different from true sleep.

FRANZ ANTON MESMER (1734-1815)

The modern use of hypnosis, however, is usually seen as originating with the German physician, Franz Anton Mesmer. Indeed, the term 'mesmerism' has become a synonym for hypnosis although Mesmer himself called his technique 'animal magnetism' and based his therapy not on the practice of the ancients but on a popular contemporary belief that magnets had the power to heal.

This theory that magnets had healing properties was first proposed in the seventeenth century by a German named Athanasius Kirchir. He maintained that a magnetic fluid ran through the body and that, if its flow was disrupted, ill health would result. (Interestingly, this is not unlike the Chinese theory of Qi or vital force which underlies the practice of acupuncture and Traditional Chinese Medicine.)

Kircher's theory was picked up a hundred years or so later by Father Maximilian Hell, a Jesuit priest and official astronomer to the Austrian court. He reasoned that, if disease was caused by a disturbance in the body's magnetic fluid, it should be possible to cure the disease by restoring the flow to normal—and the logical way of doing that would be by bringing the fluid into contact with a magnetic field. He therefore started to experiment on people by strapping magnetized iron plates to the diseased areas of their bodies.

Mesmer was a friend of Father Hell and it was through him that he started to use magnets in the treatment of his own patients. Unfortunately, his experiments with animal magnetism brought him into disrepute and it is this image of Mesmer as a quack that is the predominant one today. However, he was a qualified physician and, early on in his career, was well respected.

Mesmer came from a poor family but won a scholarship to the Jesuit University of Dillingen in Bavaria. He probably chose this university simply because the scholarship was offered, since he had no vocation for the priesthood. So at the end of his four years there, in which he studied theology, logic, metaphysics, Latin, Greek, public speaking, philosophy and science, he moved to the larger Bavarian University of Ingoldstadt. To begin with, he was enrolled in the faculty of theology but quickly abandoned the study of religion in favour of physics, mathematics, astronomy and languages.

Whether he had a voracious appetite for learning or whether he simply didn't know what he could do with what he had learned so far is not clear but, at the end of his four years at Ingoldstadt, Mesmer enrolled at the University of Vienna to study law. However, by the end of his first year there, he had transferred to the faculty of medicine and finally, in 1766 at the age of 32, he qualified as a doctor.

This was a time when many exciting scientific discoveries were being made and, for someone with Mesmer's breadth of knowledge and enquiring mind, it must have been tempting to try to link up all the new data—physical, chemical and biological. He was greatly influenced by Isaac Newton's work on gravity and believed that this newly described force must have some effect on the human body. This seemed to tie in with the idea of magnetic forces being implicated in disease and, in a paper which he wrote shortly after his graduation entitled *The Influence of the Planets on the Human Body*, he proposed that good health was dependent upon a balance being maintained between the magnetic fluid in the body and that in the external universe.

Not long after he qualified as a doctor, Mesmer married Maria Anna von Posch, a wealthy widow from an aristocratic family, who was some ten years his senior. It was her connections that enabled him to establish himself in polite society in Vienna and to set up his medical practice among the well-to-do residents of the city. And it was on a friend of his wife's, Franzl (Francisca) Oesterlin, that Mesmer first experimented with 'animal magnetism'. Maria Anna had invited her to live with them, possibly as a companion. But Franzl was not a well woman. In her late twenties, she had suffered for some two years from a whole catalogue of ailments including vomiting, toothache, earache, depression, breathlessness and fainting fits.

It must have seemed the obvious thing for Mesmer to take her on as a patient. At first, he used orthodox methods of treatment but found that, although Franzl seemed to recover for a short time, she would inevitably relapse again. This ebb and flow of the illness seemed to Mesmer like the action of a magnetic force and so he decided to treat her with the magnetic therapy that he had been reading and hearing about. His friend, Father Hell, provided the magnets and Franzl was treated. Once more, she recovered but, this time, did not relapse. Encouraged by his success, Mesmer tried the therapy on other patients suffering from similar complaints, including hysteria, depression and fits, with good results. And in the following year, 1775, he treated Wilhelm Bauer, Professor of Mathematics at Vienna University, and cured him of sleepwalking.

If Mesmer had been a poor country doctor, experimenting on the peasantry with a seemingly outlandish treatment, it is probable that he would have been left alone to continue his practice as he saw fit, perhaps being labelled as a harmless eccentric. But Mesmer's patients were not 'nobodies'—they were drawn from the aristocracy and the intelligentsia and many of them were wealthy. People began to talk about his methods and his apparent cures, and other doctors started to form their own opinions about what he was doing. Some, more open-minded than the rest, tried the magnetic treatment on their own patients. Of these, some found it helpful and continued to use it while others, whose patients showed no signs of recovery, abandoned it. The less open-minded, however, condemned it out of hand as quackery.

As with any doctor using a new and unorthodox treatment, Mesmer was aware of how important it was that the medical profession should recognize the potential value of his therapy. He therefore sent a report of his work to the Berlin Academy of Sciences, in which he put forward the hypothesis that the magnetic force involved could be communicated from one person to another and that the magnets simply acted as a channel for this. The report was studied by members of the mathematics and physics department who concluded that, although it was possible that magnetic forces could influence the human body, it was doubtful whether magnetism could be effective in producing the cures that were claimed.

So far in this story, there seems to be no apparent connection between 'animal magnetism' and hypnosis. However, all the symptoms that Mesmer was able to treat successfully were those which, nowadays, we know are susceptible to the power of suggestion. Mesmer's idea that the magnetic force was communicated from the therapist to the patient suggests that he was doing more than just strapping magnets onto his patients. As a good physician, he would have done what he could to ensure that they felt relaxed at the start of this unusual treatment and he would have explained to them exactly how he expected the magnets to work. If they were sufficiently relaxed they may well have drifted into a 'dreamy' state—and it sometimes requires only a very light trance to produce the most remarkable results.

From the beginning, Mesmer was aware that his treatment worked best when the condition being treated had been produced, or was being controlled by, the patient's mind. In some cases, such as that of a Hungarian Baron who had severe muscular spasms in his neck, he did not even use magnets but simply talked to the patient in the way that a hypnotherapist might today.

In 1775, a year after he treated Franzl Oesterlin, Mesmer was invited by the Munich Academy of Sciences to demonstrate his methods to its members and to give his opinion on a certain Father Gassner who had been curing people by the laying on of hands. Mesmer acknowledged that the Father was a very successful healer but said that he was achieving his results not, as he claimed, through exorcism but rather through the use of animal magnetism.

Looking at the way they worked, there seem to have been many similarities between Gassner and Mesmer, the only major difference being the power to which they attributed the healing. Indeed, in a paper published in the *International Journal of Clinical and Experimental Hypnosis* in 2005, Dr. Peter Burkhard claimed that Gassner's techniques were closer than those of Mesmer to the practice of modern hypnotherapy, being much more "elaborate and psychologically oriented". However, this was the Age of Enlightenment—science was in the ascendant and religion was starting to be regarded with some suspicion when it encroached on what were deemed to be scientific matters. Gassner was denounced but Mesmer was invited to become a member of the Munich Academy.

At last it seemed that Mesmer was starting to get the official recognition that he craved, and all went well until he was asked to treat Maria-Theresa von Paradies, the 18 year old daughter of the Emperor's private secretary. Although she had been blind from the age of four, Maria-Theresa was a talented pianist and, thanks to a pension granted to her by the Empress, she had been able to study with the best teachers. It seems that Dr. Stoerk, the chief court physician, was aware that her blindness was a hysterical complaint rather than a physical one, since he had treated her for several years with a variety of barbaric therapies which were used for psychiatric problems at that time, including leeches, purgatives and electric shocks to her eyes. Finally, she had been pronounced incurable by a top eye specialist. But then Mesmer took a hand in her treatment and within a month her sight started to return.

Dr. Stoerk was courteous enough to acknowledge Mesmer's success where he had failed, but other physicians were outraged that Mesmer, using bizarre methods, could cure (or claim to cure) a condition for which they had been powerless to do anything. Reports started to circulate that the girl was really still blind. And then her father, having been informed that Maria-Theresa's pension might be withdrawn if she regained her sight, demanded that the treatment be stopped.

As a result of all the stress, the improvement in the young pianist's condition could not be maintained and her blindness returned. Her father then had a change of heart and asked Mesmer to continue to treat her, which he agreed to do. It seems that she was one of the patients for whom he did not use magnets, being able to 'magnetize' (or hypnotize) her without them. After another four weeks of treatment, her sight started to return once more. But her father, probably under pressure from those who were hostile to Mesmer, would not allow her to admit that she could see, telling people that she had not been cured and forcing her to behave as though she was still blind.

In addition to all the stress that she was being put under by the politics of her treatment, poor Maria-Theresa found that, with her sight restored, her skill at the piano was diminished and, finally, she relapsed again into blindness. This, of course, gave added weight to the argument of the Viennese physicians that Mesmer was nothing but a charlatan and, as a result, the University of Vienna made a public statement to the effect that his treatment was worthless. With this condemnation, Mesmer felt that he could no longer continue to practice in his own country and he left for France.

In May 1778, Mesmer set up a clinic a few miles outside Paris, where he attracted the interest of Dr. Charles d'Eslon, who was to become a loyal patron and supporter of his work. D'Eslon was a person of some standing in the world of French medicine, being the personal physician of the Comte d'Artois—the future King Charles X of France.

Once again, Mesmer became established in the upper echelons of society and patients flocked to see him. Indeed, he had so many requests for treatment that he had to devise a method of treating more than one patient at a time. He therefore developed what he called a 'baquet'—a huge oak tub filled with water and containing iron filings and powdered glass, with phials of 'magnetized' water arranged in concentric circles. Jointed iron rods ran through the lid that covered the tub, 'connecting' the patients to the mixture within. Each patient applied one of the rods to the affected part of his or her body. Then, sitting silently round the tub, all the patients joined hands while Mesmer fixed each in turn with his eyes, waved his hands around them and touched them with an iron wand.

Around the walls of the room were mirrors which reflected carefully positioned lights; there were heavy curtains and thick carpets and, in the background, musicians played softly. Mesmer, it seems, was a master of the theatrical. But the treatment worked. His patients recovered and spread the word, so that soon, even using the baquet, he was unable to cope with the numbers who wished to be seen. In the report that Mesmer had submitted to the Berlin Academy of Sciences, he had stated his belief that any object could convey the vital magnetic fluid, not just those made of iron, and now he put that belief into practice. Attaching cords to the branches of a large tree, he asked his patients to sit holding the cords while he treated them.

But despite his undoubted success with the public, Mesmer still hankered after official approval. To try to help him achieve this, d'Eslon arranged for three representatives of the French Faculty of Medicine to visit Mesmer's clinic in order to investigate his claims. The representatives watched patients being treated but then declared that they could not make any judgement on the results since they had been unable to examine the patients personally before the therapy began. It was not the result that Mesmer had been hoping for.

In 1780, d'Eslon published a report entitled *Observation on Animal Magnetism* in which he advocated the use of the therapy. This lost him the good will of the Faculty of Medicine who accused him of using his prominent position to promote the activities of 'a German mountebank'—an interesting turn of phrase which suggests that, had Mesmer been French, the Faculty might have felt less hostile towards him. D'Eslon then suggested that a study be carried out to compare a group of patients treated by Mesmer with a group treated by orthodox methods. But the Faculty was not going to be persuaded into unbiased investigation—the suggestion was rejected and d'Eslon was told that unless he renounced his belief in Mesmer's theories within a year, he would lose his membership.

The following year, after a further unsuccessful attempt to achieve respectability and a short period spent away from Paris which had been made necessary by his despondency at its failure, Mesmer set up an organization which he named the Society of Harmony. Into this he accepted people who wished to learn about his treatment and how to use it. There was a great deal of interest and among those who enrolled were noblemen, priests, businessmen and even some doctors. In all, around 300 people received training, some of whom were then given certificates and allowed to set up their own practices, and about 40 provincial Societies of Harmony were established.

In 1784 d'Eslon, still pursuing Mesmer's dream of recognition by practitioners of orthodox medicine, managed to persuade the French queen, Marie Antoinette, to influence her husband, Louis XVI, to set up a royal commission. Five members of the French Academy of Science and four from the Faculty of Medicine were chosen and asked to investigate the therapeutic value of animal magnetism. The chairman of the commission was Benjamin Franklin, inventor, author, statesman, philanthropist and, at that time, the American ambassador to the French court. From the Academy of Science came Antoine Lavoisier, a brilliant chemist who is remembered for devising the system of atomic weights and for his work in isolating from the air the gas which he named oxygen. One of the members sent by the Faculty of Medicine was Dr. Joseph Guillotin whose name will always be associated with the instrument that was, by an ironic twist of fate, to be used to execute the deputy chairman of the commission, astronomer Jean-Sylvain Bailly, seven years later during the Reign of Terror.

The members of the commission decided, first of all, to subject themselves to treatment by animal magnetism. But when they did so, they felt nothing and therefore came to the conclusion that magnetism had no effect on healthy people. So they picked some patients to be used as guinea-pigs. However, these were not the sort of patients who would have gone to Mesmer's clinic of their own accord, and the more educated among them were sceptical about the therapy. Since antagonism to the therapy on the part of the patient makes it far less likely that hypnosis will work, the only patients who responded well were the less educated from the 'lower classes'.

After due deliberation, the commission came to the conclusion that Mesmer's cures could only be explained if either the cure or the illness was in the mind of the patient. This, of course, is a fairly crude description of hypnosis, which will alleviate symptoms that are caused or exacerbated by anxiety, tension and other negative states of mind, and which will promote 'mind over matter' to enable patients to overcome pain and other disabilities. However, in the eighteenth century, such a verdict could only mean that Mesmer was a charlatan playing on the susceptibility of gullible patients with vivid imaginations.

At the same time that Benjamin Franklin and his colleagues were deliberating, another committee, set up by the Royal Medical Society of Paris, which had not been invited to appoint members to the commission, was also investigating animal magnetism. It consisted of four members, one of whom produced a minority report in favour of Mesmer. However, the remaining three came to the conclusion that not only was his treatment useless but it could also be dangerous. Following the publication of the reports of this committee and of the royal commission, the University of Paris announced that any physician under its control who continued to use animal magnetism would have his licence to practice medicine withdrawn.

This was the end for Mesmer and he returned to Lake Constance, near his birthplace, where he spent nearly 30 years in retirement before dying in 1815 at the age of 81. However, animal magnetism did not die with him.

ABBÉ JOSE CUSTODIO DI FARIA (1756-1819) & THE MARQUIS CHASTENET DE PUYSEGUR (1751-1825)

One of those who continued to practice animal magnetism was the Abbé José Custodio di Faria, a Portuguese Catholic monk who, two years before Mesmer's death, had given a series of public demonstrations of animal magnetism in Paris. He doesn't seem to have met with the hostility which Mesmer encountered—possibly because attitudes were different in post-Revolution France or, more likely, because he was not a doctor trying to prove the value of a radical new therapy to other, more conservative, doctors.

Like Mesmer, di Faria maintained that the power of animal magnetism lay with both the therapist and the patient and that, for the therapy to be effective, both must work together. This, of course, is still true of hypnosis as it is practiced today. However, unlike Mesmer, di Faria dispensed with the more theatrical aspects—the heavy curtains, the soft music and the 'mystical' gestures. Instead, he just asked the patients to relax and to feel themselves going to sleep—a method that is very similar to that used by some modern hypnotherapists.

It was one of Mesmer's pupils, the Marquis Chastenet de Puysegur, who made the important discovery that some patients, while still 'magnetized', could open their eyes and talk. In modern hypnotherapy, it is not unusual for patients to be asked questions while they are still in a trance. Not only does this enable therapists to have a clearer idea of how their patients are reacting to the treatment but it also allows them

25

to combine other psychological therapeutic techniques with the hypnosis. While most patients are able to speak while in hypnosis, opening one's eyes without waking up — known as somnambulism — requires a particularly deep level of trance.

JOHN ELLIOTSON (1791-1868)

Mesmer's pupils, as well as continuing to practice his therapy, also taught the technique, in modified form, to others. Perhaps one of the most important of the next generation of students was an English physician named John Elliotson. The son of a chemist, Elliotson learned about animal magnetism from Richard Chenevix FRS, who had been a pupil of the Abbé di Faria, and from the Baron Dupotet de Sennevoy, who had been a pupil of Mesmer himself.

Born in 1791 in London, Elliotson qualified as a doctor at Edinburgh University and continued his studies, first at Jesus College, Cambridge, and then in London at both Guy's Hospital and St. Thomas's Hospital. From what we know of him, it seems that he was a highly skilled practitioner, but he was far more open-minded than many of the doctors of his day and his interest in new developments in medicine earned him the ridicule and hostility of others who were more conservative. He was one of the first people in England to use a stethoscope and, extraordinary as it may seem now, this was condemned by several of the top physicians of his day who maintained that this new-fangled instrument could in no way aid diagnosis.

1828 saw the opening of the new London University and, three years later, Elliotson was appointed Professor of Medicine at

University College. In 1834, he was one of three physicians to be appointed to the new North London Hospital (renamed University College Hospital in 1837). He seems to have been an enlightened teacher. In *Lives of the Fellows of the Royal College of Physicians* (commonly known as *Munk's Roll*) it is recorded that he attracted larger classes than any other teacher had done before in London. He was a "clear, precise and painstaking" lecturer, "never attempted to be oratorical or sensational" and "as a clinical teacher he was in his time unrivalled". He recognized that no two cases were exactly alike and "was gifted with singular powers of observation".

However, what distinguished Elliotson from the majority of doctors of his time was that "he accepted nothing on the ground of authority or antiquity, and rejected nothing merely because it was new; and he was ready at all times to sacrifice everything to what he believed to be truth". And this attitude, coupled with his championing of animal magnetism, was what ultimately brought about his downfall.

He had first become interested in the subject in 1829 when he attended a demonstration given by Richard Chenevix, an Irish chemist and Fellow of the Royal Society who had written a series of articles on what he referred to as 'mesmerism' in *The London Medical and Physical Journal*. However, it was not until 1837 that Elliotson began to practice mesmerism himself, after attending a series of demonstrations in which patients suffering from epilepsy were treated by Baron du Potet de Sennevoy, a French homeopath and student of the occult arts who was described by H. P. Blavatsky, author and founder of the Theosophical Society, as "perhaps the most illustrious disciple of Mesmer".

27

Elliotson was also influenced by the theories of Franz Joseph Gall, a Viennese physician and neuroanatomist who had suggested that physical disease could often be the result of the emotions acting independently of the will. However, despite his interest in the latest theories and developments in medicine, Elliotson still believed firmly in the existence of a magnetic fluid as the explanation of animal magnetism, and was also convinced that supernatural forces could be used in the diagnosis of disease.

His own early experiments with the therapy were successful and word soon got around. Medical students began to flock to his teaching sessions. But when Elliotson began to give public demonstrations of animal magnetism, the medical staff of University College Hospital were less than pleased. His final fall from grace in the eyes of the orthodox medical profession was brought about by the hostility of Thomas Wakley, the founder of the medical journal, the *Lancet*. Wakley was a qualified physician and, for a time, had been a friend of Elliotson's, supporting his experiments in animal magnetism and giving his findings wide coverage in the *Lancet*. However, the two men fell out and, in 1838, Wakley denounced Elliotson as a charlatan, based on the treatment that he had given two sisters who suffered from epilepsy.

When working with these two girls, Elliotson had used 'magnetized' nickel, since he maintained that this metal (unlike lead) was very effective in treatment. However, Wakley discovered that the two sisters responded equally well to 'magnetic' treatment when lead was used. Since Elliotson held firmly to the theory that the treatment worked because magnetic fluid flowed through the magnetized metal plates, it seemed to Wakley that the theory, and therefore the fact, of animal magnetism was now disproved. He published his findings and his thoughts in the *Lancet*, which put the authorities at University College Hospital in a very difficult position. Elliotson was asked to stop giving demonstrations and to discharge the two sisters from his care. As a result, he felt that he could no longer continue to work there and, in December of the same year, he resigned from his post.

But Elliotson did not allow the disapproval of his fellow physicians to stop him from practicing the therapy in which he believed so strongly. He founded a Mesmeric Hospital in Fitzroy Square in London, and built up a large practice there. He also started his own journal, the *Zoist*, which was mainly concerned with mesmerism and which appeared quarterly for 13 years, from 1843 to 1855. Often it printed reports which the authors had been unable to get published elsewhere because of hostility towards the subject matter. As a result of the *Zoist's* influence, several centres were established around the country for the practice of mesmerism.

The use of mesmerism to control pain formed an important part of Elliotson's work. Anesthesia was as yet unknown and patients undergoing surgery were usually tied down and given alcohol to dull the pain. The first operation in which it is recorded that mesmerism was used was the amputation of a woman's breast by a French surgeon, Jules

Cloquet, in 1829 but it is likely that other operations had been done before this.

The first operation to be performed under mesmeric trance in England was in 1842 and is recorded in *Account of a case of successful amputation of the thigh, during the mesmeric state, without the knowledge of the patient* by W. Topham (a barrister who acted as the mesmerist) and W. Squire Ward M.R.C.S. (who performed the operation at the District Hospital in Wellow, Nottinghamshire). But when the two authors read the report to the Royal Medical and Chirurgical Society of London, they were greeted with scorn and outrage, while some of the audience even suggested that the patient had been trained not to show pain. Little more was heard about the use of mesmerism in the operating theatre after this as, in 1846, conventional anesthesia was introduced.

In the same year that anesthesia was born, Elliotson was invited to deliver the Harveian Oration, an annual lecture given by a prominent physician or surgeon at the Royal College of Physicians of London. Although he had resigned from University College Hospital eight years earlier and had been publishing the *Zoist* for three years, he was obviously still respected in the medical world. Naturally, he used this prestigious invitation as an opportunity to talk about mesmerism, which probably did not go down too well with his audience of orthodox practitioners. Over the next twenty years he managed to alienate most of the medical profession and he died in poverty in 1868.

JAMES ESDAILE (1808-1859)

Of the many physicians who sent accounts of their successful use of mesmerism to the *Zoist*, perhaps one of the most significant was James Esdaile. The son of a Scottish clergyman, he was born in Perth in 1808 and graduated from the University of Edinburgh in 1830. He had suffered since childhood from asthma and chronic bronchitis and, in search of warmer climes, he took a post with the East India Company and was sent out to India. In 1838 he was appointed as surgeon to the Native Hospital at Hooghly in Bengal and it was here that he first used hypnosis in April 1845.

The patient was a man with a double hydrocele, a swelling on both sides of the scrotum. After the first side had been operated on, the patient was in severe pain. Although Elliotson had never induced a trance before, he knew how to, having read reports of Elliotson's work. So, in an attempt to relieve some of the patient's pain and thus enable the second part of the operation to be performed, he decided to try to mesmerize him. It seems as though this was a last ditch measure since he thought it unlikely that he would achieve any useful results. His knowledge of mesmerism was entirely theoretical and he had never even seen anyone use it. In addition, he was dubious about the suitability of the patient, because the ideal subject was generally thought of as being (in his words) "a highly sensitive female of a nervous temperament and excitable imagination who desired to submit to the supposed influence".

However, despite his doubts, he managed to induce a trance and to relieve the patient's pain, although it took him about an hour and a half to do so. The following day, he treated the man again and, this time, induction of the trance took 45 minutes. Five days later, when the treatment was repeated for the third time, it took only 15 minutes. The native doctors who worked with Esdaile were very impressed by the results of this *belatee muntur*, or 'European charm', as they called it, and Esdaile was inspired to try it out on other patients.

Finding that the induction of a trance was often time-consuming but that the results were well worth while, he taught his native assistants how to mesmerize the patients and used his own time for performing the actual surgery. Within eight months, he had performed 73 operations on mesmerized patients, including the amputation of an arm, three cataracts and the removal of 14 scrotal tumours weighing between eight and 80 pounds. In addition, he had treated 18 non-surgical patients whose problems included headaches, convulsions and back pain. But when he submitted a report on all these cases to the Indian Medical Board, it was not even acknowledged.

Having performed over a hundred operations successfully under hypnosis, Esdaile tried again, writing another report which he sent to Sir Herbert Maddock, the Deputy Governor of Bengal. Sir Herbert was interested enough to appoint a committee, consisting of four doctors and three laymen, to investigate Esdaile's work.

The committee came to the conclusion that it was possible to perform painless operations on mesmerized patients but thought that the method was impractical since it took a long time to produce a deep enough trance and it was impossible to predict whether or not a patient would respond. However, Sir Herbert was impressed by the fact that painless operations were even possible. He put Esdaile in charge of a small hospital in Calcutta, and appointed five physicians and surgeons as 'official visitors' to report back to him. Their findings were very favourable, and they reported that not only were patients able to undergo major operations without pain but that post-operative shock was greatly reduced.

An additional and unsolicited report was sent to the Governor General by over 300 citizens of Calcutta who had either benefited from Esdaile's treatment or had observed its beneficial effect on others. Finally, Esdaile was appointed as surgeon to Calcutta's Sarkea's Lane Hospital, where it was understood that he would combine the practice of mesmerism with orthodox medicine.

During his time in India, Esdaile performed several hundred major operations and over a thousand minor ones on mesmerized patients. Most of the major operations were to remove huge scrotal tumours which were very common in India at the time. Previously, this operation had been rarely performed because on a conscious man it had, of necessity, to be a crude and hurried affair and, as a result, about half the patients died. However, Esdaile found that with the aid of mesmerism the mortality rate dropped dramatically. While he was still in India, chloroform was introduced as an anesthetic but Esdaile was not impressed by it since, unlike mesmerism, it had many dangers associated with it.

Unfortunately, although he submitted reports of his work to the orthodox British medical journals, none of these was published since mesmerism was still looked upon with great suspicion. There was also the added difficulty that, as he was practicing so far from home, no one was able to investigate his claims. But even in India his work was not accepted by the orthodox medical fraternity and none of the Indian medical journals would accept his papers. So, as an alternative, he wrote a book entitled *Mesmerism in India*, which was published in 1850. In 1959, it was reissued by the Julian Press Inc. of New York under the title *Hypnosis in Medicine and Surgery*. It makes fascinating reading since it gives an account not only of Esdaile's experiences but also of his theories on mesmeric phenomena.

Esdaile believed firmly that mesmerism worked by the transference of a 'vital fluid' from therapist to patient and, as a result, thought that some of his success was due to the fact that his patients were usually naked and had their heads shaved. However, despite this, he also maintained that success was dependent on "passive obedience in the patient and a sustained attention and patience on the part of the operator".

Esdaile finally left India in 1851 and returned to Scotland, where he wrote another book—*Natural and Mesmeric Clairvoyance with the Practical Application of Mesmerism in Surgery and Medicine*—the following year. Once again he found himself unable to tolerate the cold Scottish climate and he moved to the south of England, where he died in 1859, aged 50.

JAMES BRAID (1795-1860)

Recognition of the true nature of mesmerism probably began with another Scotsman, James Braid, who was born in Fifeshire around 1795. Qualifying, like Esdaile, from Edinburgh University, he initially went into practice in Scotland but later moved to Manchester. A contemporary of both Elliotson and Esdaile, he first encountered mesmerism when, in 1841, he attended a series of demonstrations by a French practitioner, Charles de la Fontaine. His initial impression was that the man was a fraud and he actually went up on the stage with the intention of exposing him but, at close quarters, he found that the subject was indeed in a trance. He therefore started to experiment with mesmerism himself, using his relatives and friends as guinea-pigs.

Following the ideas of the Abbé di Faria, Braid found that elaborate ritual was not necessary and that patients could be made to go into a trance simply by making them fix their eyes on a bright object. Like Esdaile, once he had become convinced of the reality of the mesmeric trance, he entered wholeheartedly into its investigation and, within a month of his first encounter with it, he was lecturing on the subject.

In many ways, Braid's view of hypnosis was far more down to earth than that of some of his contemporaries. He rejected completely the theory of magnetic fluids, since his experiments had convinced him that mesmerism was a form of sleep. And it was he who realized that the effect of a trance was to increase the patient's suggestibility.

But, despite his more rational approach, Braid, too, found his ideas were unacceptable to the orthodox medical community. In 1842, when the British Association for the Advancement of Science announced that it was to hold a meeting in Manchester, he offered to read a paper on the use of mesmerism. However, his offer was turned down. Undaunted, Braid arranged his own seminar, to coincide with the meeting of the British Association. Many members of the Association attended and saw him demonstrate his techniques.

In the following year, he published a book entitled *Neurypnology, or the Rationale of Nervous Sleep*, in which he described "neuro-hypnotism or nervous sleep" as a peculiar condition of the nervous system which could be produced by the use of various techniques. As a more manageable term, he proposed the word 'hypnosis'.

Hypnosis, wrote Braid, would produce good or bad results according to how it was used — it was not a cure for all ills. It was, however, a powerful force and he was of the opinion that only doctors should use it and those who did not know how to use it correctly should refrain from dabbling.

AMBROISE-AUGUSTE LIEBEAULT (1823-1904), HIPPOLYTE-MARIE BERNHEIM (1840-1919) & THE SCHOOL OF NANCY

Meanwhile, in Europe, interest in hypnosis had not died. Dr. Ambroise-Auguste Liebeault read his first book on the subject in 1848, while he was still a medical student. Qualifying in 1850, he started up a medical practice in the French countryside but used only conventional methods of treatment. However, after a period of about ten years, and influenced by the work of James Braid, he once more started to study hypnosis and began to offer hypnotic treatment to his patients.

In order to ensure that he had enough subjects on whom to practice hypnosis, Liebeault offered this treatment free, only charging those patients to whom he gave orthodox treatment. Working in a poor rural area, he found that many of his patients were happy to take up the offer of free treatment, and he soon had more subjects than he could cope with.

In 1864 he moved to Nancy and set up a clinic devoted entirely to hypnosis, where he treated patients free of charge and lived off a small private income. Two years later, he published his first book, *Sleep and its Analogous States Considered From the Perspective of the Action of the Mind Upon the Body*.

In 1882 Liebeault cured a patient who had been suffering from sciatica for six years. The patient had previously been

37

treated—unsuccessfully—by Hippolyte-Marie Bernheim, Professor of Neurology at the nearby University of Nancy. Bernheim had heard about Liebeault and was deeply suspicious of the therapy he practiced. So when he heard that Liebeault was claiming to have cured this particular patient, he went to see him, determined to expose him as a charlatan. But Liebeault was able to convince him that the mind could play an important role in the development of physical illness and that hypnosis was a valid therapy to use in such cases.

Like James Braid before him, once Bernheim had been convinced of the genuine nature of the hypnotic trance, he began to investigate the therapy with a keen interest and, in 1884, he published a book entitled *De La Suggestion dans l'État Hypnotique et dans l'État de Veille* (Concerning Suggestion in the Hypnotic State and in the Waking State). In this, he proposed that hypnosis produced an increased suggestibility on the part of the patient and that it was this that caused the therapist's instructions to be effective.

Liebeault, Bernheim and their followers became known as the 'Nancy School' of hypnosis (distinguishing them from the 'Paris School' of Professor Jean Martin Charcot—see below). Their research and writings had an important influence on the work of many later physicians and psychiatrists, including Sigmund Freud.

JEAN MARTIN CHARCOT (1825-1893)

Bernheim was not the only professor of neurology who became interested in hypnosis since, until the end of the nineteenth century when psychiatry became a speciality in its own right, patients with mental disorders were usually seen by neurologists.

Jean Martin Charcot, Professor at the Salpêtrière Hospital in Paris, began to investigate the use of hypnosis in 1878. He was an important figure in orthodox medicine and his name is still known to physicians and surgeons today because of the many and varied conditions to which he gave his name—Charcot's biliary triad (signs by which a stone in the bile duct can be diagnosed), Charcot's intermittent hepatic fever (inflammation of the liver), Charcot's joints (painless deformed joints occurring secondary to another condition such as diabetes), Charcot-Bouchard aneurysms (tiny weaknesses in the walls of the blood vessels of the brain) and the Charcot-Marie-Tooth syndrome (an inherited weakness of the muscles of the legs).

Clearly, Charcot had an extensive knowledge of both anatomy and pathology, so it is somewhat surprising to discover that he subscribed to the theory of magnetic fluid and the use of magnets in the treatment of patients. His main field of investigation with regard to hypnosis was in the treatment of patients who were suffering from epilepsy and hysterical complaints. When he tried treating patients whose fits were the result of a hysterical condition, he found that not only could he remove their symptoms by hypnosis but that he could also bring those symptoms back if he gave the appropriate suggestions.

As a result of his research, Charcot came to the conclusion that only patients with hysterical conditions were hypnotizable and that hypnosis itself was a form of hysteria! Since hypnosis could be used on both men and women, the corollary of Charcot's theory was that hysteria could occur in both sexes. This was a radical idea because, until then, it had been believed that hysteria was a condition that occurred only in women and that it was caused by a displacement of the womb (the word hysteria being derived from the Greek word *hystera*, meaning 'womb').

HYPNOSIS AND PSYCHIATRY

A great deal of work in the field of hysterical complaints was carried out by the Viennese physician Dr. Joseph Breuer (1842-1925) who put forward the theory that hysterical symptoms were often the result of the patient having experienced some sort of trauma. He developed the technique of regression which allowed the patient to re-experience the previous trauma and, by fully expressing the emotions associated with it, get it out of his system. His work had a great influence on the young Sigmund Freud (1856-1939), with whom he worked and who, for some time, was a keen practitioner of hypnosis.

Freud qualified as a physician from the University of Vienna in 1881 and won a scholarship to undertake further studies in the department of neurology at the Salpêtrière Hospital in Paris. It was here that he met Charcot and was introduced to hypnosis and to psychology. He started to use hypnosis himself in 1887 and it was this that led him to develop his own technique of psychoanalysis.

It was Freud who coined the term 'catharsis' (from the Greek word *katharsis* meaning 'cleansing') to describe the technique of releasing suppressed emotions that had been pioneered by Breuer. Ultimately Freud abandoned hypnosis in favour of free association and, as the medical profession became increasingly interested in psychoanalysis, hypnosis became less and less popular in psychiatric practice.

HYPNOSIS IN THE UK—1890s TO PRESENT DAY

By the end of the nineteenth century, the orthodox medical profession was beginning to change its attitude towards hypnosis. In 1891 the British Medical Association set up a committee to look into the phenomena that it could produce, its value as a therapy and "the propriety of using it". The following year, the committee produced a unanimous report in which it was agreed that the hypnotic trance was a genuine state comprising "altered consciousness . . . increased receptivity of suggestion from without . . . [and] an exalted condition of the attention" and in which the patient was susceptible to post-hypnotic suggestions. (A post-hypnotic suggestion is one which is given while the patient is in a trance and which takes effect after he or she has woken up.)

The report commented on the fact, often re-stated since, that the term 'hypnosis' was somewhat misleading, since it implied that it was a form of sleep. It acknowledged, however, that the therapy was often effective in "relieving pain, procuring sleep and alleviating many functional ailments". It pointed out that there was danger in "want of knowledge, carelessness or intentional abuse" and reiterated James Braid's recommendation, made 50 years earlier, that only doctors should be allowed to practice the therapy. It also expressed strong disapproval of public exhibitions of hypnotism and recommended that these should be restricted by law. However, despite the continuing concern of doctors, public exhibitions of hypnotism are still allowed more than a century later.

During the First World War, a large number of casualties suffered from what was then called shell shock and which we now refer to as post-traumatic stress disorder or PTSD. Army psychiatrists were inundated with work and were happy to use anything that would speed up the patient's recovery. This led to a resurgence of interest in hypnosis. And practitioners were now starting to find other uses for hypnosis, in addition to the treatment of purely psychiatric complaints.

The use of hypnosis for dental extractions, in place of anesthesia, was probably pioneered by James Milne Bramwell (1852-1925) a Scottish surgeon whose interest in the therapy began when he was a child. His father, Dr. J. P. Bramwell, had seen demonstrations given by Esdaile who, at that time was working in Scotland, and his enthusiasm had communicated itself to young James. In time, James followed his father into the medical profession and, while training at Edinburgh University, was particularly interested by lectures given by the physiology professor, John Hughes Bennett, on the work of James Braid.

Once qualified, Bramwell went into general practice and started to use hypnosis for himself. In 1890, at a meeting in Leeds, he demonstrated hypnotic anesthesia to a medical audience. Both the *British Medical Journal* and the *Lancet* carried reports of the meeting and, as a result, Bramwell had so many patients referred to him that he had to abandon his general practice and concentrate solely on hypnosis.

It was the use of hypnosis as an anesthetic that made it so useful in dental treatment where, for minor procedures, a general anesthetic seemed unwarranted. (Local anesthetics for dental procedures only started to be developed in the early years of the twentieth century.) On some occasions Bramwell was present and hypnotized the patient before the dentist started work. But with other patients he used the technique of post-hypnotic suggestion. While they were in hypnosis he would tell them that, when they were in the dentist's chair, if a certain phrase should be repeated to them, they would immediately go into a deep trance. Then all he had to do was to write to the patient's dentist telling him which phrase to use and how to wake the patient up at the end of treatment, and the patient could be hypnotized every time he went for dental treatment.

However, dentists proved to be just as hard to convince as physicians had been and it was a considerable time before the use of hypnosis in dentistry became acceptable to more than just a few. The first sign that attitudes might be changing was probably the publication, in 1938, of a paper in the *British Dental Journal*—the journal of orthodox dentistry. The author of the paper, Eric Wookey, (1891-1985) suggested that hypnosis could be of use to prevent pain during scaling, fillings, extractions and minor oral surgery, and that it would also help to alleviate any fear or pain that the patient was experiencing before the treatment began.

Wookey said that he had accumulated convincing evidence that hypnosis could be of real value in pain relief. He was also of the opinion that it could promote rapid healing and prevent haemorrhage, although proof of this was harder to obtain. By writing the article, he hoped to induce his colleagues to take up the study of hypnosis so that their combined experiences could be used for the benefit of the dental profession. However, it was another 14 years before this came about.

Interest in hypnosis was also growing within the medical profession and, in 1949 Dr. Sidney J. Van Pelt, an Australian physician working in London, founded the *British Journal of Medical Hypnotism*, remaining its Editor in Chief until it ceased publication in 1966. Van Pelt was the first full time medical hypnotherapist in London and, in addition, was a prolific writer, publishing eight books on hypnosis between 1953 and 1960. But although he was able to bring together the top names in hypnosis, who contributed to the *Journal*, he met with continuing hostility from the orthodox medical profession, and detailed proposals that he put forward for teaching hypnotherapy to doctors were not taken up.

In 1952, an Essex dentist, Harry Radin, proposed the setting up of a committee of dentists to study hypnosis. Eric Wookey was appointed chairman and, the committee evolved into the British Society of Dental Hypnosis. This heralded a sudden burst of publicity for dental hypnosis. It started when a demonstration of a dental extraction under hypnosis at the annual meeting of the British Dental Association was reported widely and in extravagant terms by journalists who still equated hypnosis with hocus pocus. Just two weeks later, the BBC current affairs program *Panorama* showed another dental extraction under hypnosis, and this resulted in even greater press coverage.

The following year, a sub-group of the Psychological Medicine Group Committee of the British Medical Association was appointed to look into the use of hypnosis in medicine. It reported that the sort of phenomena that were observed when a patient was in hypnosis shed a great deal of light on the workings of the unconscious mind. It found that hypnosis was of use in surgery, obstetrics and dentistry and suggested that it might even be the treatment of choice for some psychosomatic and psychiatric illnesses. It recommended, therefore, that medical students should learn about hypnosis as part of their psychiatric training and that courses should be available for anesthetists and obstetricians. However, more than half a century later, hypnosis is still taught mainly in post-graduate courses and is a closed book to many anesthetists and obstetricians.

It was not until the early 1960s that the press began to write about hypnotherapy in terms that recognized its scientific basis and its valuable practical applications. But within the medical profession, interest was growing. In 1955, the British Society of Dental Hypnosis became the Dental and Medical Society for the Study of Hypnosis, amalgamating in 1961 with a group of doctors who were practicing hypnosis to form the

Society for Medical and Dental Hypnosis (later becoming the British Society for Medical and Dental Hypnosis).

In 2007, the British Society of Medical and Dental Hypnosis amalgamated with the British Society of Experimental and Clinical Hypnosis to form the British Society of Clinical and Academic Hypnosis (BSCAH) whose aim is "to promote the safe and responsible use of hypnosis in medicine, dentistry, and psychology, and to educate both our professional colleagues and the public about hypnosis and its uses". It runs training courses, like the BSMDH before it, and membership is open to all health professionals.

HYPNOSIS IN THE USA

The first person to try to bring animal magnetism to America was a Frenchman, the Marquis de Lafayette. He had been one of the founder members of the Parisian Society of Harmony, which Mesmer had set up in 1782. Both Lafayette and Mesmer wrote to George Washington who was politely non-committal. When Lafayette visited America, he gave a few lectures but it seems that he was unable to stir up much interest.

In 1829, Joseph du Commun, a French mesmerist who had emigrated to the USA, gave a series of lectures in New York but, like Lafayette, had little success in converting his listeners.

Five years later another Frenchman, Charles Poyen St. Sauveur (died 1844), who had encountered mesmerism when studying in Paris, arrived in the USA where he worked, to

46

begin with, as a teacher of French and drawing. His interest in mesmerism led him to begin work on a book (published in 1836 as *Report on the Magnetical Experiments*) and to give lectures which, at first, met with indifference. However, in Rhode Island he started to attract more interest and was able to find an excellent subject, Cynthia Ann Gleason, whom he took with him on his subsequent tour of New England, which included a demonstration at Harvard Medical School. He published his second book, *Progress of Animal Magnetism in New England* in 1837.

Contemporary reports suggest that, rather than being serious academic lectures, Poyen's demonstrations had more than a passing similarity to modern stage hypnosis, with some of his subjects giving demonstrations of clairvoyance while in a trance. However, before long, he had started to acquire pupils and, in 1836, one of these, B. F. Bugard, wrote to the *Boston Medical and Surgical Journal* to say that he had painlessly extracted a rotten tooth from a twelve year old girl while she was under hypnosis.

Another of Poyen's pupils was Phineas Parkhurst Quimby (1802-1866) who gave up his job as a watchmaker in order to become an itinerant lecturer on mesmerism. One of his patients was Mary Baker Eddy, the founder of Christian Science, and it has been said that Quimby's belief that the mind plays a major role in the development of disease influenced her philosophy.

The number of practitioners of mesmerism grew steadily. One who drew huge audiences for his demonstrations was

Robert Collyer (1814-1891), an Englishman who had studied with John Elliotson. Having arrived in the USA in 1838, he was particularly active in Boston, where an investigation by the city council, although not going so far as to endorse hypnosis, declared that it was neither dangerous nor a fraud. Collyer also experimented with the use of hypnosis as a painkiller, testing it against ether and opium, and developed his own metaphysical theory on how the therapy worked.

Another demonstrator who drew huge audiences was John Bovee Dods (1795-1872) who was already an established lecturer on his theory of 'electrical psychology'—the belief that electricity was "the connecting link between mind and inert matter". From this, it seems that it was just a short step to mesmerism. In Lecture One of his *Six Lectures on the Philosophy of Mesmerism: Reported by a Hearer*, first published in 1847, we read that he had been invited to speak by "several distinguished members of both branches of our legislature" and that this lecture was attended by "more than two thousand hearers". The first edition of the book, comprising 3000 copies, was sold out within a month of publication.

Another major figure in the world of hypnosis at this time was La Roy Sunderland (1804-1885), a Methodist minister who believed there was a strong similarity between a hypnotic trance and a state of religious ecstasy. He called himself a 'pathetist' rather than a mesmerist and rejected the 'magnetic fluid' theory of hypnosis, believing instead that all hypnotic trances were self-induced and derived from the suggestibility of the subject. In the journal, the *Magnet*, which Sunderland produced intermittently between 1842 and 1844, 'pathetism' is described as signifying "susceptibility, to passion, emotion or feeling, of any kind, produced by manipulation, and that agency, also, by which any effects of this kind are produced on the mind, or physical system".

Sunderland's emphasis in his journal was on the medical use and investigation of hypnosis and he described numerous cases in which it had been used in a therapeutic way. He disapproved of "public exhibitions of the magnetic sleep". They were, he wrote, "liable to serious and insurmountable objections; and many of them, we know, have done much to bring the subject of Magnetism into disrepute". People who knew about hypnosis had never approved of "persons traveling about the country, carrying subjects with them, or when they attempt to operate for mercenary purposes . . . The wonder is not, merely, that any person of good character could adopt such a method for making money, but that any should be found willing to be operated on in this way". Sunderland would find himself in agreement with a number of present-day medical hypnotherapists.

Gradually, interest in hypnosis spread to other parts of the country and, particularly in small towns which didn't have recourse to more sophisticated medicine, it started to be used to induce anesthesia for operations and dental extractions, although once anesthetic drugs became more widely available, the use of hypnosis was abandoned.

In the 1930s, however, a psychologist named Clark Leonard Hull (1884-1952) started to research into hypnosis and its medical uses, including the control of pain. His experiments showed that the hypnotic state is much more akin to the waking state than it is to sleep, and Hull suggested that the only major difference between hypnosis and the waking state was the degree of suggestibility. Unfortunately, when he took up a position at Yale medical school, he was forced to give up his research as a result of the school's concern regarding its safety. His book *Hypnosis and Suggestibility*, based on his findings, was published in 1933.

Also investigating hypnosis in the first half of the twentieth century was the psychiatrist and psychologist Milton Erickson (1901-1980). A prolific writer, and first president of the American Society for Clinical Hypnosis, Erickson was a controversial figure who developed techniques whereby a seemingly normal conversation or a handshake could be used to induce a hypnotic trance. He investigated ways of working with resistant patients and techniques by which a trance could be deepened. Although some of his writings have been challenged by other researchers, his work had a major impact on the establishment of hypnosis as a valid therapy.

Around the middle of the twentieth century, two hypnotists were working hard to train doctors, dentists, psychologists and psychiatrists around the USA. Interestingly, neither came from a medical background. Dave Elman (1900-1967) had been a stage hypnotist but, having seen the value of hypnosis in relieving the pain of his father who was dying from cancer, he eventually decided to teach hypnosis where it could do most good. He traveled widely around the USA for over a decade and, in 1964, published *Findings in Hypnosis* (renamed in later editions *Explorations in Hypnosis* and then *Hypnotherapy*).

Harry Arons (died 1997) was a research scientist and writer who taught hypnosis for 40 years and demonstrated to the legal profession how hypnosis could be used in a forensic context. He was the founder of the Association to Advance Ethical Hypnosis and the author of several books, including *Hypnosis in Criminal Investigation*.

While, thanks to Elman and Arons, the techniques of hypnosis were being more and more widely used, Ernest Hilgard (1904-2001), who was professor of psychology at Stanford University, was undertaking research into the therapy. Together with Dr. André Muller Weitzenhoffer, he developed the so-called Stanford scales for assessing an individual's susceptibility to hypnosis. His book *Susceptibility to Hypnosis* was published in 1965.

By the second half of the twentieth century, hypnosis was generally accepted as a valuable therapy. The American Medical Association approved its use in 1958 (although encouraging further research) and the American Psychological Association followed suit in 1960. Hypnosis was also being used by the legal profession, to help witnesses to recall details.

A major figure in forensic hypnosis (that is, hypnosis used in a legal context) around this time was Professor Martin Orne (1927-2000) who demonstrated conclusively that it was possible for a hypnotist to induce a subject to 'remember' things that had not actually happened. Towards the end of the century, his ideas fuelled the arguments over false memory syndrome. However, although some of his ideas were controversial, his academic standing was such that his championship of hypnosis helped it to continue to gain ground as an accepted psychological technique.

CHAPTER THREE: PSYCHOSOMATIC ILLNESS—THE EFFECT OF THE MIND ON THE BODY

The circumstances in which hypnotherapy can be of value can be divided roughly into three groups: those in which there is need for pain control (such as dentistry and obstetrics), those in which the patient is suffering from an emotional or mental problem (such as anxiety, phobias and some types of insomnia) and those in which the patient has a psychosomatic condition.

Now, 'psychosomatic' is a greatly misunderstood word, since people often believe it to mean that the disease is 'all in the mind'—in other words, that the patient is just imagining the symptoms. But people who are suffering from psychosomatic disorders know full well that their symptoms are real. Patients who imagine that they are ill are hypochondriacs—and that's something completely different.

New York University's Professor John Sarno's dictum "The pain is real, but the cause of the pain isn't" sums up psychosomatic pain—an area in which he is a respected expert. He believes that, in many cases, the body creates physical pain in order to draw the mind away from painful emotional issues which are deeply buried in the subconscious mind. By helping the patient—using psycho-education or psychotherapy—to acknowledge this and to deal with the mental distress, the physical pain can be cured.

In psychosomatic illness, the body and the mind both play a role and, indeed, the derivation of the word, from the Greek *psyche* meaning 'mind' and *soma* meaning 'body' implies that the two components are equally involved in the disease process. Hypnotherapy, of course, only treats the mind but is effective because it can relieve the stress or emotional trauma which has either caused the condition or is making it worse. Research has shown that the sympathetic nervous system, which regulates the 'fight or flight' reaction to danger, is affected by stress and, as a result, the body will behave as though it were constantly facing danger, with raised blood pressure and heart rate and an increased production of hormones from the adrenal glands. Stress can also interfere with the body's immune mechanism, making the subject more susceptible to infection and to inflammatory conditions.

Among the commonest psychosomatic conditions (that is, conditions where the patient's mental state has either created or is exacerbating the problem) are high blood pressure, asthma, migraine, impotence, psoriasis, eczema and digestive disturbances.

Peptic ulcers (duodenal and stomach ulcers) used to be considered the epitome of psychosomatic illnesses. The condition was seen predominantly among people who were in stressful jobs or who had constant anxieties. However, it was then discovered that some 80 per cent of these ulcers were caused by a bacterium called helicobacter pylori. So why was the condition so prevalent in people who were stressed out? Further research demonstrated that only one fifth of all those who have helicobacter in their digestive tracts actually develop ulcers—but that stress greatly increases the chances of them doing so. Here, then, was a perfect example of physical and mental components working together to cause illness.

Another condition where physical and mental factors work hand in hand is asthma. At root, asthma is a physical condition. The bronchi (the small airways in the lungs) are more sensitive than normal, so that contact with any irritant, such as pollen, house dust or animal fur, may cause them to constrict and to secrete sticky mucus, making it harder to breathe. This is a frightening condition, so the patient's anxiety may increase dramatically and this can cause further constriction and worsening of the symptoms. Indeed, many patients who suffer from recurrent asthma will get an attack if they become stressed or anxious. A vicious cycle is set up, with the asthmatic attack and the anxiety feeding on each other. If the patient is taught a method by which to calm the anxiety, the attacks are likely to occur less frequently and be less severe.

Many bodily processes, such as breathing, occur automatically, without us having to think about them. But if we do start to think about them and to worry about them, it can interfere with normal functioning. It is not uncommon for insomnia to occur in this way. Most of us have the occasional sleepless night—possibly because we're worried about a problem. Once the problem has been resolved, the chances are that we'll start to sleep normally again—unless we've started to worry about the fact that we've not been sleeping. And, if that's the case, it becomes a vicious cycle—

anxiety about insomnia causing more sleepless nights which, in turn create more anxiety.

A similar situation can occur in men who experience an episode of impotence. This is not an uncommon condition and it will happen to most men at some time or another—perhaps because they've had too much to drink or just because they're over-tired. Whatever the reason, it probably won't still be affecting them next time they want to have sex. Most men realize this and accept the temporary failure as just that—temporary. But sometimes a man—perhaps unable to understand why he should have failed on this particular occasion—will start to worry about it so that next time he will be aware of a nagging anxiety in the back of his mind that he may not be able to get an erection. And, if the anxiety becomes too great, this in itself may prevent him from having an erection. In the same way that anxiety can set up a vicious cycle of insomnia, it can do exactly the same with impotence. The answer in both cases is to understand what is happening and let go of the anxiety (helped, perhaps, by some hypnotherapy or psychotherapy).

It can be hard for people in the West to understand how much the body can be affected by the mind because Western medicine tends to treat patients as though they were a loose collection of relatively unconnected parts: a patient with a mental illness is referred to a psychiatrist, someone with arthritis is seen by a rheumatologist, and a patient with appendicitis will come under the care of a surgeon. This is quite different from the holistic viewpoint of most complementary and Oriental therapies.

The term 'holistic' is derived from the Greek word *holos*, meaning 'whole', and a practitioner of holistic medicine will treat the patient as a whole, and not as individual and unconnected parts. If a woman comes in complaining of arthritis, for example, the holistic practitioner will want to know not just about her joints but also about how the rest of her body functions, about her anxieties and concerns, her work, her home life, her social life, what she eats, what exercise she gets, her hopes and ambitions, her sleeping patterns and so on. These are things that make up the individual patient and, if she is ill, they may all contribute to that illness or be affected by it.

THE NERVOUS SYSTEM AND ITS ROLE IN PSYCHOSOMATIC ILLNESS

While complementary therapies may have their own theories as to why body and mind are so firmly interlinked (for example, the theory of acupuncture talks about the Qi or life force which flows round the body) Western medicine demonstrates the connection through a study of physiology and biochemistry.

If you were to study the anatomy of the human body, it would soon become clear that, although different parts (such as the kidneys and the tongue, or the lungs and the feet) seem totally unlike each other, there are two things that they have in common. The first of these is a blood supply which every part of the body (apart from the hair and nails which are made of a dead substance called keratin) needs in order to remain alive and functioning. The second is a nervous system.

The most complex part of the nervous system is the brain, which is responsible for all the 'higher' functions such as thinking, memory, speech, hearing and sight. But many simpler functions are carried out through the spinal cord, an extension of the brain which runs down inside the hard protective cover of the bones of the spine, or vertebrae. Together, the brain and spinal cord form what is known as the central nervous system, or CNS. Because these two parts of the CNS have separate roles, a broken back may cause paralysis without affecting any of the 'higher' functions such as memory and speech, while someone with severe brain damage may still retain some normal bodily activities.

Both brain and spinal cord are made up of very delicate tissue and both have to be protected—the brain within the skull and the spinal cord within the vertebral column. The nerves, however, have to leave this protected environment and run out into the body where they can receive messages and send back signals from the CNS which tell the body how to function. This 'exterior' part of the system is known as the peripheral nervous system (or PNS).

The head, its special sense organs (eye, ear, nose and tongue) and the neck are supplied by the cranial nerves which come directly from the brain. One of these, the vagus, travels further than the others and has an important role in the functioning of the throat, voice, stomach, intestines, heart and lungs. The spinal column is made up of 24 separate vertebrae which are joined to each other by ligaments and muscles (allowing the spine to move and to bend). At the top end, the spine is connected to the skull and at the lower end to the pelvis. Where a vertebra joins its neighbour, two nerves leave the spinal cord, one going to the right side of the body and the other to the left. These nerves then divide many times to form a vast network which supplies the entire body.

Although we think of nerves as being continuous, solid cords, they are, in fact, made up of huge numbers of tiny fibres which interact with each other, rather like the numerous tiny fibres that go to make up a piece of rope. When a message travels down a nerve, it takes the form of an electrical impulse. However, where two nerve fibres meet, there is a tiny gap, across which the impulse cannot pass. So when it reaches the end of a fibre, it causes a chemical (known as a 'neurotransmitter') to be released and this stimulates the next fibre to pass the electrical impulse along its length.

Research into the production and action of neurotransmitters has enabled modern Western medicine to develop drugs that exert some control over the nervous system. For example, some of the muscle relaxants that are given to patients undergoing major surgery act by preventing the release of a neurotransmitter that carries a message telling muscles to contract.

In terms of its function, the nervous system is divided into two sections, the somatic (or voluntary) and the autonomic (or involuntary). We have, of course, already met the word 'somatic', meaning 'bodily', in the term 'psychosomatic'. The autonomic nervous system, as its alternative name implies, functions automatically and controls all the bodily actions that we don't have to think about consciously, while the somatic nervous system is in charge of voluntary action such as walking. In order to walk, you must have a conscious wish to do so. You don't suddenly find yourself strolling down the street when your intention was to sit down and read a book.

However, you don't have control over basic bodily functions such as the beating of your heart and your breathing (unless you are a very highly developed yogic practitioner). This means that you don't have to remember to keep breathing and you don't have to remind your heart to beat or your stomach to digest your food—which is just as well! This, obviously, means we can get on with living our lives. But it does have a down side. It means that we have to trust our autonomic nervous systems to work normally. If you bend your leg and it hurts your knee to do so, it's a relatively simple procedure to unbend it again to relieve the pain. But if the autonomic nervous system malfunctions and starts to increase your heart rate, for example, it's less easy to get it back to normal.

The autonomic nervous system is divided into two parts—the sympathetic and the parasympathetic whose functions, in a healthy person, will balance each other out, since they work in opposite directions. As a result, the heart will beat neither too slowly nor too fast, the stomach will produce the correct amount of acid to digest the food presented to it, and the breathing will continue at a normal rate.

So why do we need two opposing systems to regulate these basic body functions, rather than one? Well, every now and again, our bodies need to adapt to changing circumstances. For example, when we run or take other strenuous exercise, the sympathetic nervous system increases the respiration rate and the heart rate so that an increased amount of oxygen is delivered to the muscles, to enable them to work. It also stimulates the liver to release glucose into the bloodstream to give the muscles energy. Then, when the exercise is at an end, the parasympathetic system will bring the body back to its resting state.

It is likely that this balancing act developed originally so that early human beings (and animals) could protect themselves from predators and, although the dangers facing people in the modern world are, on the whole, far less life-threatening than those faced by early man, our sympathetic nervous systems react in exactly the same way. If we're going for an important job interview, taking an exam, about to go on stage to act in a play or give a speech, we still react with the same 'flight or fight' response, even if these reactions are totally inappropriate to the actual situation.

When the sympathetic nervous system is stimulated, the pupils of the eyes widen (to ensure that we see every movement around us), the tiny muscles attached to the base of each hair contract so that the hair stands on end (very useful if you're a small animal trying to pretend that you're bigger and fiercer than you actually are), the heart rate speeds up (so the body is supplied with as much oxygen as possible), the arteries supplying blood to the heart muscle dilate so that the heart can work harder, and the muscles in the airways relax so that air can go in and out rapidly and easily. In addition, the blood vessels supplying blood to the digestive tract and any other functions that, for the time being, are not essential, are constricted so that increased amounts of blood can be sent to the limbs (whose blood vessels are dilated) thus preparing the body for either fighting or running away.

In a true 'fight or flight' situation, the exercise of fighting or of running will maintain the blood pressure, even though there is considerable dilation of the blood vessels in the limbs. However, if neither fighting nor running away is appropriate (for example, if someone with a needle phobia is about to have a blood test), then the dilated vessels may result in a sudden drop in the blood pressure and a feeling of faintness. And while all this is going on, the sympathetic nervous system is also stimulating the sweat glands to release sweat. This is why someone who has had a severe shock may look pale and sweaty and feel faint.

Meanwhile, the adrenal glands are busy pumping adrenaline into the blood stream. The adrenal glands lie just over the kidneys and go into action in response to fright, shock or excitement. This is why many of the symptoms of fear and of excitement—'butterflies' in the stomach, shortness of breath, a rapid heart rate, trembling—are so similar. Probably the major difference between fear and excitement is the person's state of mind—happy and positive (excitement) or anxious and negative (fear).

If you're feeling excited, the surge of adrenaline can be quite a pleasant experience. Top athletes rely on that feeling before a race to give them the will to win. Similarly many actors and singers will admit to 'nerves' before going on stage and know that this will help to keep them on their toes and give a good performance. The 'nerves' usually disappear as soon as a performer steps onto the stage but, if they have been excessive, more adrenaline will have been produced than is needed and the 'nerves' will continue and interfere with the performance. It's exactly the same with exam nerves — the student who is slightly nervous and 'keyed up' beforehand is likely to do better than either the student who has no emotions or the one who is very agitated.

If you watch wildlife programs on television, you'll know that animals living in the wild tend to have periods of rest interspersed with episodes when they are either tracking and killing prey or having to fight to defend themselves. In other words, their autonomic nervous systems are stimulated perhaps three or four times a day but, in between, they will return to a normal balanced state. However, it's different for many human beings nowadays. Despite the fact that we're not built to be in a constant state of stimulation, that's the way that many of us live. We have stressful jobs, we drive in heavy traffic, we're frequently in a rush, we watch horror movies, we listen to the news, we argue with our family and friends . . . the list goes on and on. And, as if this were not enough, we stimulate our bodies to produce even more adrenaline and other hormones by smoking, eating large amounts of sugar and junk foods, and drinking coffee and alcohol, while our autonomic nervous systems are trying to keep our bodies functioning normally.

It is little wonder, then, that stress, anxiety, smoking and poor eating and drinking habits can lead to illness. The balance cannot be maintained and the body will either stay in a constant state of sympathetic-type anxiety (ready to fight or flee) or the parasympathetic system may become overactive if the sympathetic has exhausted itself.

THE ROLE OF HYPNOSIS IN PSYCHOSOMATIC DISORDERS

An imbalance between the two parts of the autonomic nervous system may be at the root of many psychosomatic disorders and there is no doubt that stress and anxiety can exacerbate many conditions which, initially, have a physiological or pathological cause. So if one can bring the patient's autonomic system back into balance, control of the disease will be easier. There are, of course, measures that can be taken to prevent excessive stimulation—for example, eating and drinking sensibly, stopping smoking and keeping calm. But while most people, when needs must, will be able to reform their diet and drinking habits and to stop smoking, staying calm if you have a naturally anxious temperament is easier said than done.

However, this is where hypnotherapy comes into play because it is, first and foremost, a very effective relaxation technique. When you go into hypnosis, your body—and your mind—realize that they do, after all, know how to relax. In addition to this, suggestions can be given that you will be less tense and less anxious in your everyday life. So not only will you feel calmer overall but this calmness will help to control whatever problem it is that is affecting you.

So, for example, hypnotherapy is widely used for the treatment of asthma, migraine, irritable bowel syndrome, eczema and psoriasis—all of which have a tendency to get worse if the patient becomes anxious or stressed. Psychosomatic illness can be seen as a vicious cycle, with anxiety being a vital component. Removing the anxiety will break the cycle and allow the body's own defence mechanisms—which, up till then, have been fighting a losing battle—to take over and restore the patient to health.

Even today, no one is entirely sure how hypnosis works in relation to the brain and nervous system. Scientific experiments have been able to demonstrate that the state of hypnosis exists but actually identifying what occurs in the brain to make that happen has proved more difficult. Mostly, hypnosis is defined by what it does rather than by what it is. The Mayo Clinic says it is "a trancelike state in which you have heightened focus and concentration" while the British Medical Association calls it "A temporary condition of altered attention . . . in which a variety of phenomena may appear spontaneously or in response to verbal or other stimuli". Dave Elman (see chapter two) stated that "Hypnosis is a state of mind in which the critical faculty of the human is bypassed, and selective thinking established", while Sigmund Freud commented (in his article *On Psychical Treatment*) that "hypnosis is in no sense a sleep like our nocturnal sleep or like the sleep produced by drugs. Changes occur in it and mental functions are retained during it which are absent in normal sleep."

What most, if not all, definitions agree on is that in hypnosis patients are open to suggestions that things are different from the way they really are and will accept these suggestions uncritically. So patients who are in pain can be told that the pain is disappearing and they may indeed be aware of this happening. Or, as sometimes occurs in stage hypnosis, a subject is handed a piece of apple and is told that it is an onion, and his eyes start to water just as though he were smelling an onion. In other words, his autonomic nervous system, which controls automatic reactions such as crying, is responding to what the subject believes. It is, so to speak, the other side of the coin from the man who cannot get an erection because he believes it won't happen and therefore it doesn't. The man with the phoney onion believes it will make his eyes water and therefore it does.

Experiments in which hypnosis has been used to control allergic responses show how very strongly our beliefs affect the way in which our bodies react. One of the most impressive is that carried out by two Japanese researchers, Yujiro Ikemi and Shunji Nakagawa, who published their report, *A Psychosomatic Study of Contagious Dermatitis*, in the *Kyushu Journal of Medical Science* in 1962. Their subjects were a group of high school students who were allergic to the leaves of two related plants — the Chinese lacquer tree (Toxicodendron vernicifluum) and the Japanese wax tree (Toxicodendron succedaneum). If any of these students came into contact with the leaves of one of these trees under normal conditions, their skin would become inflamed at the point of contact.

Under hypnosis, the students responded to contact with these leaves in the same way that they usually did. However, the experiment was then repeated and they were told that the toxic leaf with which one arm was being stroked was

66

something to which they were not allergic. Then the other arm was stroked with a chestnut tree leaf (to which they would not normally react) and they were told that it was one of the toxic leaves. Amazingly, the skin stroked with the chestnut tree leaf became inflamed while that stroked with the toxic leaf showed little or no response.

Other researchers have demonstrated similar results. The mind, it seems, can control the autonomic nervous system to such an extent that it is capable of allowing tiny blood vessels to dilate and fluid to seep out of them (as happens in an allergic reaction) in a small and fairly sharply delineated patch of skin.

Experiments such as these show very clearly the effect of hypnosis on the automatic functions of the body. But how the hypnotic state actually occurs is more difficult to say. It is, for example, quite easy to determine whether or not someone is asleep by looking at an electro-encephalogram (or EEG) which shows the electrical activity going on in the brain. But there seem to be no specific changes in someone who is in hypnosis. His heart rate and respiration rate may slow down and his blood pressure drop, as is likely to happen in anybody who is sitting comfortably and completely relaxed. But the EEG will show the same pattern that it would if he were awake. While he is going into hypnosis, it will show the slow so-called alpha wave patterns that occur if one sits quietly with eyes shut and thinks of nothing. And when the hypnotherapist starts to make suggestions for the subject to think about, the EEG will show that the brain is thinking, just as it would if he were awake.

In an article published in 2001, Solomon Gilbert Diamond and Robert D. Howe of the Harvard University Division of Engineering and Applied Sciences wrote "Clinical hypnosis is a mindbody technique that operates at the intersection of subjective perceptions and objective physiological changes. A fundamental problem with hypnosis research is that the subjective mental state of patients during hypnosis cannot be measured directly." In order to determine whether a failure to respond to hypnotic treatment was due to the treatment not being effective or whether it was simply because the patient was not in hypnosis, it was necessary to rely on the patient's subjective opinion.

Diamond and Howe proposed a method of monitoring the depth of a hypnotic trance by measuring the variability in the heart rate between subsequent beats of the heart (HRV). They pointed out that "The heart rate exhibits spontaneous fluctuations even at rest that reflect the continuous influence of the autonomic nervous system". The experiment was designed to discover if there was "A single parameter [that] can be calculated from HRV that will change systematically during the hypnotic state when compared with a control condition that is commensurate with the hypnotic state". Their results suggested that it might, indeed, be possible objectively to measure the depth of a hypnotic trance in this way. A further study, by Diamond, Howe and Orin C. Davis, published in the *International Journal of Clinical and Experimental Hypnosis* in 2008, confirmed their original findings.

But while it may now be possible to measure the depth of a hypnotic trance, there is still no clear indication of why hypnosis works as it does. It has been suggested by some researchers that a hypnotic induction in which the patient is asked to concentrate hard on a single thing may cause his brain to become less aware of the other stimuli that normally impact on it—smells, sounds, pain, tastes, feelings and so on. The continuous, monotonous speech of the hypnotist may then reduce this awareness still more until all the patient is aware of is this speech.

However, how can one explain the fact that while under hypnosis the patient's subconscious mind is so much more accessible than normal? This, after all, is the reason why post-hypnotic suggestions work—they are planted in the subconscious and the patient obeys them automatically, without having to think about them, and sometimes without even being aware of them. In addition, the subconscious can reveal what is troubling it far more readily and old suppressed memories and emotions can be brought to the fore and dealt with.

It has been suggested by a number of investigators that these effects of hypnosis are due to the differences in function of the left and the right sides of the brain. Anatomically, the two sides of the brain are, to all intents and purposes, identical, with the right side receiving messages from the left side of the body and the left side receiving messages from the right. This is why a stroke caused by a blood clot in the right side of the brain will affect the left side of the body; if the clot occurs in the left brain, then the right side of the body will be affected. However, if the paralysis is on the right (with the damage in the left brain) there is a much greater chance of the patient's speech being affected than if the paralysis is on the left. This is because, despite their similar anatomy, the two sides of the brain don't function in exactly the same way.

The left half of the brain controls speech and logical thinking but the right side is much more concerned with the emotions, creativity and intuition. And because language is a function of the left brain, a patient whose left brain is incapacitated and whose right brain is functioning alone, while knowing what to do with a knife and fork, will accept uncritically the information that they are called 'a cup and saucer'.

These discoveries have led to the theory that, when a patient is under hypnosis, the logical left side of the brain relaxes and allows the right side to come to the fore. This would explain the ability of the patient, under hypnosis, to bring out long-repressed memories (the repression being a function of the left side of the brain) and to accept uncritically whatever suggestions are put to him, since these would not appear to be illogical.

CHAPTER FOUR: HYPNOSIS AS THERAPY

IS IT GOING TO HELP?

Most people who have been hypnotized will have found it a very pleasant and relaxing experience. Indeed, many are reluctant to come out of the hypnotic state at the end of their session, in the same way that they might be reluctant to wake up from a pleasant dream in a warm comfortable bed when they know they have a busy day ahead.

Before waking a patient from hypnosis, the therapist will usually tell him that when he comes out of the trance he will feel relaxed, happy, free of pain, or whatever is appropriate to the situation. So the patient, who has been sitting in an extremely relaxed state for half an hour or so, may start to feel the benefit of the treatment as soon as he opens his eyes. With some patients this benefit is only small at first. But others may say that they feel that a weight has been lifted from their shoulders or that they are feeling more relaxed than they have done for a long time.

However, it must be stressed that, in order for hypnotherapy to help you, you must *want* to get better since it is, first and foremost, a self-help therapy. It will help you to do what, in your heart of hearts, you want to do. Sometimes, though, people will have reasons, locked in their subconscious minds, for not wanting their condition to improve. Such patients are unlikely to feel much benefit from their sessions unless, somehow, this unwillingness to get better can be discovered and brought to the attention of the conscious mind during hypnosis.

It may seem strange that there are patients who want to remain ill but this may happen, for example, in the case of a person who has done something for which, subconsciously, he cannot forgive himself and for which he is punishing himself. It may also happen if the patient is getting actual benefit from the illness, such as increased attention or not having to face up to responsibilities. This latter situation is known as secondary gain and needs to be distinguished from that of the malingerer who pretends to be ill in order to gain an advantage. In secondary gain, the illness is quite real and stems from an attitude of the subconscious mind.

The majority of patients, fortunately, have no such problems and are anxious to get better. And, for them, a hypnotherapy session is likely to be a comfortable and relaxed period from which they may derive a definite—and often an immediate—benefit.

AM I HYPNOTIZABLE?

If you've been thinking about having hypnotherapy, you may have wondered whether you'd be a 'good subject', and doubts about this may have been putting you off trying it. Obviously, if you don't think you can be hypnotized, there's little point in going to see a hypnotherapist.

Because hypnosis is a natural state, it's quite rare for people to be completely unhypnotizable—and, when it happens, it's usually because they've either been resisting or else they've been so anxious about whether or not they'll 'go under' that their anxiety has stopped the hypnosis from working. Many patients are amazed at how readily they go into a hypnotic trance, even on their first session.

In fact, most people have been in a light hypnotic trance many times in their lives. The commonest way to go into hypnosis naturally is to daydream. Most people know what it is like to go into a vivid daydream, where you lose all sense of time and of your actual surroundings. And when you 'wake up' from the daydream, it is sometimes a shock to find that you're not in the place that you were imagining. This vivid kind of daydream is, in fact a form of self-hypnosis. And that is why people with vivid imaginations are usually good hypnotic subjects—they have had lots of experience!

HYPNOSIS AND MEDITATION

Some types of meditation also induce a form of hypnotic state, particularly those in which a word or phrase (*mantra*) is repeated over and over again. This is a meditation technique that many people have found useful in relieving anxieties and tension, allowing them to develop a more positive outlook on life, and helping to control conditions related to anxiety, such as eczema and irritable bowel syndrome.

It would be wrong, however, to assume that all types of meditation induce a hypnotic state. The term 'meditation' can mean different things to different people, and meditation techniques are many and varied. The Buddhist system

73

of mindfulness of breathing is, for example, completely unrelated to hypnosis because, although the practitioner focuses on the breath going in and out, his aim is not to concentrate on that to the exclusion of all else but, rather, to focus his mind perfectly while remaining totally aware of everything that is going on around him.

The purpose of Buddhist and various other forms of meditation is to increase the spiritual awareness of the practitioner, and an interesting distinction between this form of meditation and hypnosis has been made by some healers who claim to have observed the different effects of each upon the aura, or psychic energy, of the individual. The aura, they say, grows larger in people who meditate regularly, being particularly noticeable during the act of meditation. (Legend says that the Buddha had an aura that was three miles wide.) But when a patient is put into hypnosis, say the healers, his aura retracts inwards. In other words, the psychic energy and the 'higher functions' of the mind are temporarily shut down, while the deeper, subconscious mind opens up.

More scientifically, the differences between meditation used to increase spiritual awareness, the 'hypnotic' types of meditation, and hypnosis itself may be demonstrated by wiring subjects up to an electro-encephalograph (EEG) machine and measuring their brain waves. Those who are sitting, relaxed with eyes shut, or who are in hypnosis, or who are practising a 'hypnotic' type of meditation will show a pattern of slow 'alpha' waves on the EEG, interspersed with rapid 'beta' waves that appear whenever they are spoken to or asked to think about something. A constantly repeated short noise will produce, to begin with, a short burst of beta waves each time it is heard. But, after a while, the brain will grow accustomed to the sound and will, so to speak, screen it out, so that it no longer registers on the EEG.

When the meditation is geared towards spiritual development, however, the result is quite different. William Johnston, in his book *Silent Music* (Collins 1977), describes an experiment in which experienced Zen meditators were wired up to EEG machines while they sat in meditation. It was found that, unlike the 'hypnotic' meditators, their brains never grew accustomed to anything. No matter how often a particular sound was repeated, each time they heard it, their brains reacted as though they were hearing it for the very first time.

THE DEPTH OF THE TRANCE

Various techniques have been developed to try to determine how deep a trance patients have achieved. One of these, devised by the American psychologist Leslie M. Lecron (1892-1972), consists of asking subjects to assess their depth, on a scale of nought to one hundred, while they are in trance. The problem with this is that it requires a measure of concentration on the part of the subject and this, in itself, may lighten the trance.

Other systems consist of asking subjects to do something in hypnosis (such as losing sensation in one finger or temporarily forgetting a particular piece of information) and then assessing how readily they are able to do this.

While some patients feel that they go deeply into trance, it is not uncommon (particularly after a first session) for someone to question whether he was actually in trance. Some are only eventually persuaded that they *have* been hypnotized by the fact that the therapy is starting to work!

Some patients are concerned because they tend not to go very deeply into trance but, in fact, this doesn't usually matter very much. There are some forms of treatment, such as age regression, where a deeper trance is needed in order to achieve results—and certainly patients do seem to respond better to suggestions if they are in a deeper trance—but this does not mean that hypnotherapy will be unsuccessful for a patient who can only achieve a light trance. Indeed, there is plenty of treatment that can be carried out with only a very light trance and, although the condition may take longer to resolve if the patient is unable to go deeper, it is still perfectly possible to achieve good results from hypnotherapy. So don't worry about whether or not you are likely to be a 'good subject'. It is the results of the treatment that are important, not the depth of the trance.

THE HYPNOTHERAPY SESSION

The training that aspiring hypnotherapists receive differs from institution to institution so there is no such thing as a 'standard' session. The information in this section is based on my own hypnotherapy training (with the British Society of Medical and Dental Hypnosis) and my own practice.

A first session will usually last about an hour (unless you are seeking help to stop smoking, in which case it may be shorter). The therapist will take a full case history and will want to know about the problem that has caused you to seek treatment, whether anything makes the symptoms worse or better, and your attitude to the problem (in other words, whether it's making you anxious or depressed or whether you tolerate it with good humour). He will also ask you about your home circumstances, your job, your lifestyle and any other anxieties or worries you may have.

There are two reasons for all these questions—firstly, it will help the therapist to discover the cause of the trouble and, secondly, it will enable him to express himself in a way that your mind will readily accept when he gives you post-hypnotic suggestions. For example, if you suffered from migraine and your attack always started with little dots of yellow light swimming in front of your eyes, followed by a numb feeling in your mouth, the therapist, knowing this, can tell you, when you are in hypnosis, that these specific symptoms will not occur. This is far more effective than just telling you that you will no longer get migraine.

Similarly, if you find something helpful in alleviating your symptoms—for example, if you have a skin condition and a particular cream helps to stop the itching—you might be told that performing a certain action (such as taking a deep breath or clicking your fingers) will relieve the itching in exactly the same way that the cream does. In this way, you have something within your own experience to which you can relate the therapist's suggestion and this makes it more likely that it will be effective.

On the first occasion that you are hypnotized, you may only go into a very light trance. This may be because you are slightly apprehensive about the therapy or anxious that you may prove to be unhypnotizable. By the second session, these anxieties should have dispersed and you are likely to be more relaxed and receptive to the treatment.

The methods used to induce a trance are many and varied, and different practitioners have their own favourites. Usually they are fairly simple and consist of you being asked to focus hard on something—an object, an action or a feeling—while the therapist continues to talk to you.

Once you're in trance, there are various methods that can be used to deepen it. One is to ask you to imagine a soft, warm light flowing over you and gently helping your muscles to relax by soothing away any tensions. Another is to ask you to imagine that you're in a beautiful garden. Gradually, everything in the garden becomes very clear, so you can see the individual flowers, smell the roses, feel a light breeze on your cheek, and hear the birds singing. This is just an extension of the 'vivid daydream' mentioned earlier. By asking you to use more than one of your senses—sight, smell, feeling and hearing—the therapist is helping you to lose yourself in the visualisation. This will allow you to become more relaxed so that the trance will deepen.

Another technique that is sometimes used in conjunction with a visualisation, such as the garden, is to ask you to picture some steps that go down to a lower level. You are then asked to walk slowly down the steps—and, as you do so, the trance gradually becomes deeper and deeper.

Imagining downward movement is a very effective way of deepening a trance and, for those patients who don't suffer from claustrophobia and who don't mind traveling in lifts, visualizing a downward journey in a lift can increase the depth considerably.

One 'lift' technique is to ask the patient to imagine that he is in a lift that is descending from, say, the fifth floor. At each floor, the lift stops and a certain number of people get in and get out, so that each journey from floor to floor acts as a separate deepening technique. Finally, the lift goes into the basement—"the basement of relaxation"—and the patient visualizes himself getting out, moving into a warm, softly lit room, and sinking down into a comfortable armchair. However, the therapist really needs to have his wits about him if he is using this method, or the patient may finish up no deeper in trance than at the start.

One therapist told me about an occasion when he used this technique, saying to the patient "We are now at the fourth floor and two people get out and one gets in . . . we are now at the third floor and one person gets out and one gets in . . ." and so on, without concentrating on the numbers he was using. However, when he got to the basement and asked the patient to relax in the armchair, he had the impression he wasn't any deeper in trance than when he had started. So, when he woke him up at the end of the session, he asked whether he had found it hard to picture the lift. "Not at all,"said the patient. "I could see the lift clearly. The problem was that, by the time we got down to the ground floor, we had minus six people in there!"

Because the patient was struggling to follow the therapist's instructions in his visualization, it was interfering with his ability to go deeper into trance. The images used in deepening have to be both soothing and relaxing. So, obviously, the lift technique wouldn't be suitable for someone who suffered from claustrophobia. And it might not be sensible to ask a patient who suffered from severe hay fever to imagine taking a stroll through a garden at the height of summer.

Sometimes you may be asked to pick your own visualization —whatever you find relaxing—perhaps a walk by the sea or in the countryside or through a wood. One of the most important things about this type of visualization is that you see yourself as the only person there. If you're on a beach, it should be deserted (apart, perhaps, from the odd sea bird) and not one on which people are packed like sardines. For children, however, it is sometimes helpful to let them imagine that they have a trusted adult with them—perhaps a parent or even the therapist.

Not all deepening techniques require visualization. For example, the therapist may count to ten, or to twenty, synchronizing his counting with your breathing, and telling you that, as the count continues, you will become more and more relaxed. Or he may ask you to take a very deep breath, hold it for a few seconds and then let it out very slowly, feeling, as you do so, that you are sinking down, deeper and deeper into trance. Yet another method is for the therapist to pick up your arm, holding it loosely by your sleeve, and tell you that, when he drops the arm gently back into your lap, it will act as a signal for you to go even deeper into trance.

Your arm can also be used in a method called hand levitation. There are several variations of this, but in all of them you will find your arm rising into the air as though of its own accord. In one version, you are asked to imagine a balloon bobbing above your head. The string is tied to your wrist and you can feel a gentle upward tug. Gradually your arm lifts up, pulled by the balloon. Because you are already in a light trance and therefore in a suggestible state, you will usually be able to picture and feel the balloon, and your arm will start to rise.

There may be a problem, though, with the more scientifically minded patient who is aware that an air-filled balloon could not possibly tug his wrist upwards, and who is not yet in a deep enough trance to be able to accept this suggestion uncritically. This is why some therapists may mention, in passing, that the balloon is filled with helium—a gas that is lighter than air!

Once you have pictured the balloon lifting your arm, the therapist will tell you that the string is going to be cut and your arm will fall gently back into your lap. And you will be told that, as your hand touches your lap, this will be a signal to go even deeper into trance. Because this method is a combination of visualization and the 'signal' technique, it may help you to go into a deeper trance than either one used alone.

Most hypnotherapists' treatment rooms are quiet and comfortable but you can never predict when there might be a sudden intrusive noise—a 'phone ringing or a helicopter flying overhead. However, any extraneous noises can be put to good use and, far from detracting from the level of the trance, can actually add to it. This is achieved very simply by the therapist telling you "If, while you are in hypnosis, you hear any sounds other than my voice, you will take them as a signal to go even deeper asleep".

'EGO-STRENGTHENING'

Once you are as deep in trance as the therapist considers necessary, the treatment proper begins. Since most conditions which respond to hypnotherapy involve some degree of anxiety and self-doubt, the technique of ego-strengthening is widely used and forms an important part of the treatment for many patients.

Ego-strengthening consists of certain suggestions given by the therapist concerning the way you feel about yourself. At a very basic level it may just consist of the therapist telling you that you will feel more confident and self-assured and will be able to cope better with your life. Or visualizations may be used. One that is used by some therapists is to get you to visualize a large round blob, which is identified as a human egg, and to see many, many sperm swimming towards it, looking like tadpoles. You are asked to identify with one sperm and to watch it as, swimming very strongly, it pulls ahead of the others and, reaching the egg first, fertilizes it. As it does so, you are asked to feel the sense of achievement that comes with winning a race and are reminded that this is the way your life began—with the best sperm fertilizing an egg. The very first event in your life was a triumph so, having proved yourself capable of success by winning that race, there is no reason why you should doubt your capabilities in other directions.

Another ego-strengthening technique is to ask you to remember some incident when you really felt pleased and satisfied with yourself and to project yourself back to it. You are told that you will remember exactly how you felt on that occasion and will be able to relive your pride in your achievement. Once you have indicated that you are, indeed, feeling that satisfaction and pride, you will be asked to do something physical, such as clenching your fist or rubbing your fingers together, and you will be told that whenever you repeat that movement you will be able to recapture that same feeling of achievement. So, if at any time you are feeling low or unsure of yourself, you will be able to use this technique to boost your self-confidence.

Some people, while being able to cope well with their normal routine, find that certain situations cause them to feel nervous or to lose confidence. Here visualization may be very helpful in enabling the patient to picture himself confronting such situations with assurance. For example, let us suppose that the patient is a man who holds a responsible position in a large company. He enjoys his job and is good at it but, from time to time, he has to give lectures, which he dreads. Having to stand up and speak in public terrifies him but, because he doesn't have to do it very often, it hasn't affected the rest of his work. However, he is aware that, because of his fear, the standard of his lectures is poor, no matter how well he prepares them, and he always spends a miserable week in a state of nerves before each lecture.

In such a case, the patient may be asked, once he is in hypnosis, to imagine himself going about his normal work, and then to see himself doing one thing extremely well and being congratulated by his superiors. This would be followed by a suggestion that, because he knows that he is very capable in his everyday work, this feeling of confidence will remain with him through the session of hypnotherapy. He is then asked to see himself going into the lecture room, with his notes in his hand. Gradually, he imagines himself giving the talk, still retaining the feeling of confidence. The therapist may direct his attention to the members of the audience, who are listening attentively and are obviously enjoying his lecture. When he has finished, they all applaud enthusiastically, boosting his confidence still further.

The great advantage of visualizing a stressful situation under hypnosis, as opposed to experiencing the real thing, is that, should the patient start to feel anxious, the scene can be 'frozen'. His feeling of confidence is then built up once more before the visualization is restarted. Once he has pictured himself giving a lecture a number of times and has remained confident throughout, it will start to become easier for him to do so in real life. A technique such as this would normally be used in conjunction with other forms of ego-strengthening.

Usually ego-strengthening techniques are given at the start of a hypnotherapy session and are followed by treatment directed towards specific complaints. (Chapter seven looks at individual complaints and how they might be treated.) In addition, some other more general techniques may be taught. For example, you may be told that if, when you're in a stressful situation, you repeat a certain phrase to yourself (such as "calm and relaxed"), you will feel your anxieties and tensions disappear. Or you may be taught to imagine that you are surrounded by an invisible but protective barrier that you can put up at any time to prevent yourself from being upset by other people or by difficult situations.

While hypnosis increases the suggestibility of the subject, visualization is a very powerful technique by itself. One valuable version of the 'barrier' technique which will work even if you haven't learned it under hypnosis, is to imagine yourself wearing a long cloak made of dark blue velvet. It pulls snugly round your neck, goes right down to your feet and overlaps in front, covering your entire body. The hood pulls up over your head, leaving just your face uncovered. The cloak is lined with a light silky material and the cloak itself is very roomy. Inside the cloak is your own inner space which cannot be invaded by anyone else. The cloak can thus protect you from the 'outside world'.

SELF-HYPNOSIS

During the first session of hypnosis, or sometimes the second, you may be taught how to hypnotize yourself. Self-hypnosis can be a vital part of the treatment for many patients. Normally, you will only see the therapist once a week or once a fortnight and, in between the sessions, it is the self-hypnosis that keeps the treatment going. It's like the practice that you need to do if you're having piano lessons— the more you practice, the better you become.

And so you may be asked to set aside about 20 minutes a day to put yourself into hypnosis. During this session you can practice the various relaxation techniques you have learned, or use relaxing visualizations such as imagining yourself walking in a garden or lying on a beach, or you may be given specific visualizations to use, connected with the problem that is being treated. For example, the man who was scared of lecturing might be asked to picture himself giving a lecture while remaining relaxed and comfortable.

There are two methods by which you can put yourself into hypnosis. Some therapists like to make a recording of the session and give you the CD to listen to at home. In this case, your self-hypnosis practice will be identical to your session with the therapist. The second method is more flexible, with the therapist giving you a post-hypnotic suggestion that a certain series of words or phrases, when you repeat them to yourself, will have the effect of putting you into hypnosis. Doing it this way enables you to concentrate on whatever you think is most necessary on any particular occasion, and allows you to make the practice session as long or as short as you wish.

The series of words or phrases used to induce self-hypnosis is always unconnected (for example "sleep . . . practice . . . one, two, three, four, five"). It is never a single word or a single phrase which might come up in conversation and which might, if you are particularly susceptible, result in you going into hypnosis at an inappropriate moment. And, because it could be dangerous to go into hypnosis under certain conditions, other precautions also need to be taken, whichever method you are given.

These precautions take the form of suggestions, given to you while you're still in hypnosis. You will be told that you will only be able to go into trance in circumstances where it's safe for you to do so. (I had one patient who found self-hypnosis very easy and who, on one occasion, while having a long relaxing bath, decided to put himself into hypnosis. But he found that he couldn't, because his subconscious mind knew that it wasn't safe to be hypnotized while lying in the bath.)

Having been taught how to put yourself into a trance, you will be told how to wake yourself up. You will also be told that, if anything happens while you're in a self-induced trance that needs your immediate attention, you will wake up straight away and be fully alert to deal with it. The emphasis here is on something that needs immediate attention, rather than just something that you are aware of but that is not urgent. So, for example, if you were to smell burning, you would automatically wake up. But if the telephone rings, you can decide whether or not you want to wake up and answer it.

These precautions are, of course, absolutely essential to your safety and their inclusion or omission by a therapist who teaches self-hypnosis may give an indication of how well-trained that therapist is. Hypnosis is a very easy technique to learn—anyone can put someone else into a hypnotic trance. Unfortunately, if you don't know what to do with it or how to control it, it can become a very dangerous technique, so it is vital that you go to a therapist who has had adequate training. (See chapter nine for advice on how to find a therapist.)

Self-hypnosis is perfectly safe if you have been taught by a qualified therapist, since he will not allow you to do anything that might cause you harm. If you are hypnotized by a doctor, dentist or psychotherapist, he may tell you, while you are still in trance, that you will not allow yourself to be hypnotized other than by a medical professional. Other properly trained therapists will use a different form of words, but the intention is the same—to prevent you from being hypnotized by someone who has no knowledge of what might occur once you are in trance, and no training in how to deal with it.

CHAPTER FIVE: THE THORNY QUESTION OF STAGE HYPNOSIS

The subject of stage hypnosis is a controversial one. There is a large body of people (mostly doctors and those who believe that they or their loved ones have suffered as a result of stage hypnosis) who would like to see it banned because they think it is dangerous. Indeed, as long ago as 1892, a special committee of the British Medical Association that had been set up to investigate various aspects of hypnosis expressed its "strong disapprobation of public exhibitions of hypnotic phenomena, and the hope that some legal restriction would be placed upon them". However, there are also people (including, of course, those who make a living from putting on stage hypnosis shows) who say that it is perfectly safe. And there are others who believe that, while it shouldn't be banned, certain safeguards are essential.

The trouble is that it is well-nigh impossible in many cases actually to prove that it was the hypnosis that was responsible for the problems encountered by volunteers after the show had finished. A case in point is that of Christopher Gates who was described as an easy-going, placid man, dedicated to his job—before he volunteered as a subject for a well known stage hypnotist. Within days of the show, Christopher's behaviour had started to change and became increasingly bizarre. He was admitted to hospital, where he was diagnosed as having acute schizophrenia.

Four years later, Christopher took the hypnotist to court, claiming £250,000 in damages. The court heard that there was no family history of mental illness, and an eminent psychiatrist who had treated him stated that he believed the condition had been triggered by the hypnosis and that "There is nothing to indicate he suffered schizophrenia for any other reason". Despite this, however, the judge dismissed the claim—and the psychiatrist's evidence—saying "It is highly improbable that the onset of schizophrenia has anything to do with his participation in the hypnotism show".

This is contrary to the views of many doctors and psychiatrists —and also of ex-stage hypnotist Jeremy Wheeler who writes on his website *The Dangers of Stage Hypnosis* that, in his opinion, "If a person is bordering on psychosis then hypnosis can be the trigger that fires them into insanity".

But, of course, there is no way of proving this. We have no way of knowing whether, had Christopher Gates not volunteered as a subject, he would have remained free from schizophrenia, or whether it would have happened anyway, in response to some other trigger.

Because of this uncertainty, very few stage hypnotists have been successfully sued by their unhappy subjects. One case that was successful, though, was that brought by Ann Hazard, a 25 year old woman who, while on stage under hypnosis, needed to go to the bathroom. The hypnotist, told her to use the quickest exit. Because people in hypnosis tend to take instructions at face value, Ann took what she perceived to be the quickest route—and walked straight off the edge of the stage, breaking her leg. The injury was a serious one, requiring her to undergo surgery so that metal plates and pins could be inserted and a bone graft performed. Previously, she had enjoyed running and judo but the accident meant that she could no longer do either of these.

Because there was no doubt in anyone's mind that her injury was the result of a careless instruction while she was in a trance, she was awarded damages—but only against the theatre where the show was held. As a newspaper report pointed out, there would have been no point in her suing the hypnotist himself, since he was uninsured.

The matter of insurance is an important one. Unless stage hypnotists are fully regulated by law, they cannot be forced to take out insurance to compensate any subject who sustains an injury. In recent decades, professional bodies of stage hypnotists have been founded in order to try to maintain higher standards and these bodies do require all their members to be insured. For example, in the UK the Federation of Ethical Stage Hypnotists (founded in 1979) has a code of conduct to which members must adhere. This includes regulations about appropriate advertising, who can be used as subjects, and what safeguards must be used. But, of course, membership of organisations such as the FESH is not compulsory, so there are still many stage hypnotists who are not bound by any rules.

In the UK, stage hypnosis is governed by the Hypnotism Act of 1952. Despite two later attempts to make it tighter by introducing amendments, it still doesn't have much in the way of teeth. While the act makes it illegal to use subjects under the age of 18, there is no restriction on what the hypnotist can do with his subjects. However, in some other countries such as Israel and Norway, and also in a few states of the USA, hypnosis can only legally be used by doctors and psychotherapists who are fully trained and qualified to do so.

It has to be said, however, that hundreds of thousands of people have volunteered to be subjects for stage hypnotists over the years and have suffered no ill effects. It would seem, reading the various reports available, that the majority of problems have arisen in people who have been very good subjects and have gone into a deep trance. But it's not unknown for others—and indeed for members of the audience too—to be affected. In 1952, when the UK Hypnotism Bill was under consideration by Parliament, a 'summary of expert opinion' compiled by the National Association for Mental Health stated that "there is some evidence in respect of people in [the] audience who have not been stage volunteers, subsequently suffering unpleasant and worrying symptoms which can be directly attributed to witnessing such performances". And ex-stage hypnotist Jeremy Wheeler states that "On numerous occasions I have had members of the audience fall into trance, and even follow the suggestions given to the participants on stage".

Clinical psychologist Frank Machovec, in his book *Hypnosis Complications: Prevention and Risk Management* lists many frequently reported side effects of stage hypnosis, including headaches, anxiety, fatigue, dizziness, disturbed sleep, disorientation, and difficulties with memory and concentration. He also maintains that post traumatic stress disorder and even death may occur.

One case where it was claimed that stage hypnosis was implicated in a death was that of Sharron Tabern, a 24 year old British woman, who died within hours of volunteering to be a subject for a stage hypnotist. At the autopsy, it was found that her death had been caused by her inhaling vomit while she was asleep . . . but there was no indication as to why she should have vomited (she had only had a small amount of alcohol during the course of the evening) nor why her cough reflex (which normally should have prevented this) was not working.

One interesting—and unexplained—finding was that the amount of the hormone prolactin in Sharron's blood was 14 times the normal level. Levels are known to rise after epileptic seizures and also as a reaction to stress. It was suggested that Sharron may have had a fit—but, once again, there seemed no reason why this should have happened.

However, it was suggested by Sharron's friends and family that what had occurred during the hypnosis show would have caused her considerable stress. She had had no reason beforehand to believe that this might be the case—in fact, she had told her family and friends that she was excited about going to see the show and intended to volunteer.

An investigation of the case by Australian psychotherapist and hypnotherapist, Tracie O'Keefe, comes to the conclusion that Sharron would have been a very good subject and likely to go deeply into trance. Not only was she enthusiastic about being a volunteer, but she was also known to be very imaginative and very trusting—both attributes which would have made her more suggestible. Another factor was that she had not needed any anesthetic while giving birth to her two children. William S. Kroger (1906-1995), an American obstetrician who was a pioneer in the medical use of hypnosis, commented in his book *Clinical & Experimental Hypnosis* that women who are able to go through labor without anesthetic have a natural ability to go into a deep trance state.

During the show, Sharron was given suggestions which may seem distasteful—she was told she could see all the men in the audience in the nude, and she was told to kiss a man in the audience (who she probably didn't know). But it was only at the end that something occurred which her family and friends were certain must have stressed her enormously. According to a witness, the hypnotist told Sharron that he was going to wake her up and, as she woke, she would feel 10,000 volts of electricity coming through the seat of her chair—and it would hurt.

Now, as I have already said, someone who is in a deep trance will accept what is said to her at face value. Most people will become stressed if they are told they're going to experience pain. But, in Sharron's case, there was an additional factor. She was terrified of electricity. When she was 11, she had touched an electric wall socket and had received a shock which had blown her across the room. She had never recovered from the fear this caused and, as an adult, would not even change a light bulb. Added to this, a few weeks before she volunteered as a subject, her father had received an electric shock—fortunately not fatal, but serious enough for him to sustain burns and have to take time off work.

So what must Sharron have felt when she was told that she would feel a massive electric shock? Fear? Terror? I have mentioned before that a hypnotist cannot make someone do something they don't want to do (such as give up smoking when they really have no wish to), but the electric shock was not something that Sharron was told she would do—it was something that she was told would happen to her. She was also told that it would happen in conjunction with 'waking up' out of hypnosis. It is possible (although unprovable) that her subconscious mind tried to protect her by stopping her from 'waking up'. True, she was observed to jump out of her chair when the hypnotist counted to three to wake her, but the friends who were with her on that night said that, after the show finished, she complained of a headache and dizziness and she didn't seem to be fully connected with what was going on. It is possible that she was still in a trance.

This would mean that the suggestion that she would feel 10,000 volts when she woke was still active—still waiting to happen. Having gone to sleep, she may then have experienced the shock when she woke up after a few hours. Whatever the cause, by the next morning she was dead.

The verdict of the coroner at the inquest into Sharron's death was that she had died from 'natural causes'. Sharron's family disagreed. They applied for leave to appeal to the British High Court against the verdict. This was refused on the grounds that the case consisted simply of one set of theories against another—in other words, neither side had any proof to support its case. The judge who ruled on the appeal also commented that, even if the hypnosis had been a contributory factor in Sharron's death, the coroner was still correct to bring in a verdict of 'death by natural causes'.

In her paper on the case, Tracie O'Keefe writes "It is my opinion that [the judge] failed to comprehend the gravity of his decision in that it now gives the impression that stage hypnotists are allowed carte blanche to practice their art, and should someone be injured, the stage hypnotist may not necessarily be held accountable."

Of course, not all complaints against hypnotists are as serious as this. Thankfully, cases such as Sharron's are very rare. However, it is not unusual for lesser complaints to hit the headlines, particularly if the hypnotist involved is well-known.

In 1951, less than a year before the UK Government passed the Hypnotism Act which forbids the use of subjects under the age of 18, Margaret Proctor, a 14 year old Scottish girl, and her two 16 year old friends volunteered to take part in a stage hypnotism show. After the show, one of the 16 year olds kept falling into a trance. After three weeks, during which she was said to have done this more than 50 times, she was taken to hospital where a medical hypnotherapist was able to treat her. Margaret felt sleepy after the show and kept falling asleep, even while she was walking along. She, too, required hospital treatment. The third girl suffered from severe headaches and kept lapsing into trance every time she heard a particular tune.

It seems clear, even after all this time, that the hypnotist failed to remove a suggestion (about feeling sleepy or falling into trance) that was given during the performance and, possibly, did not take adequate steps to ensure that all his subjects were awake at the end of the show. This is a point addressed in the code of conduct of the FESH (which, of course, wasn't to come into being for another 28 years). It states "I will ensure that any hypnotic or post-hypnotic suggestions are removed completely before any subject leaves the room . . . [and] towards the end of each performance I will give specific suggestions to all subjects and to members of the audience that they should awake and, on awaking, they should feel fit and that they should not go to sleep again until they retire to bed in the normal way".

Another headline-making case in which, it seems, a suggestion may not have been removed was that of the British woman Diana Rains-Bath. In March 1952, only months before the Hypnotism Act passed into law in the UK, she sued the hypnotist Ralph Slater for negligence and assault. Slater was an American citizen but had spent his childhood in England. He was a popular stage hypnotist on both sides of the Atlantic but, in the 1940s, had been in trouble with the authorities in the USA when he marketed a gramophone record which he claimed could cure insomnia.

Diana caught his show when he was performing at the Brighton Hippodrome in 1948. She was 19 years old. Like Sharron Tabern, she was a naturally deep subject and she was one of the three volunteers who Slater picked out from an initial 15 or 20 to use in the show. Once she had been hypnotized, he is reported to have said to her "You will do just what I tell you." It is possible that Diana was resistant to this suggestion because, when Slater moved to work with another of the volunteers, she woke herself up. Slater immediately came back to her and forced her head forwards, commanding her to sleep. Diana reported later that she was aware of pain as he did this, and it was on this that the charge of assault was based.

When she was again in trance, Slater told her that her chair was getting hotter and hotter so that she could no longer sit on it—and, as a result, she jumped up. He also said that, after she woke up, if he stamped on the floor, she would get up from her seat and shout "Peanuts"—which he got her to do, after she'd returned to the audience. This, of course, was all fairly harmless stuff. A little later on, though, Slater told Diana that she was going to be like a little baby that was frightened and crying for its mother. And, indeed, she did start crying and calling out "Mummy! Mummy!". As this was not a suggestion that would have felt threatening or would have gone against her moral principles, it's not surprising that, being a good subject, she complied with it.

And all would probably have been well, but for the fact that Slater didn't remove the suggestion of feeling frightened and wanting her mother before he woke Diana up. When she awoke she said she felt tired and dazed, although this soon passed off. However, a week or so after the show, she woke up one morning feeling frightened, depressed and tearful. During the trial she told the court "My mind seemed miles away and I couldn't concentrate on anything." Although the depression lifted, it was only temporary, and she continued to have periods of depression, each longer than the one before.

Diana consulted several doctors and, eventually, was referred to Dr. S. J. Van Pelt who, at that time, was President of the British Society of Medical Hypnosis. He was an ardent advocate for the regulation of stage hypnosis and it may well be that Diana's case was a powerful influence on his views. He treated her for a period of four months, after which the depression had lifted and any residual effects of the hypnotic suggestion seemed to have been removed.

In court, Dr. Van Pelt stated that the manoeuvre in which Slater forced Diana's neck forward would have interfered with her circulation and blood pressure and could have been dangerous. He also gave it as his opinion that "It is a foolish thing to tell anybody [to feel frightened and cry for her mother] because crying brings along with it deep fundamental emotions which have a great effect on the mind and such suggestion could cause much harm".

In his defence, Slater told the court that he had learned hypnotism by studying and practicing. (In other words, he was self taught.) He said that he had been giving public demonstrations for over 15 years and had hypnotized well over 25,000 people (including using "mass hypnotism by radio") and had never previously had a claim made against him as a result of a hypnotic demonstration.

Diana's counsel, John Flowers, referred to Slater's book *Hypnotism and Self-Hypnosis* (published in 1950) in which he

99

had written that hysterical people should not be hypnotized. How, Mr. Flowers wondered, could Slater ensure that none of the people who had listened to him on the radio had a hysterical temperament—or, for that matter, any of the 20 or so strangers who came up on stage at every performance?

The jury was in no doubt that Diana's condition had been precipitated by the hypnosis and found Slater guilty. He later appealed against the verdict. The Court of Appeal decided that the original judge had omitted certain facts in his summing up and, in light of this, while allowing the verdict concerning the assault to stand, dismissed that concerning the negligence and ordered a retrial. Interestingly, no retrial was ever staged because the Government (in the shape of the Home Office) told Slater to leave the country.

Nowadays, hypnotists in the UK who are members of the FESH agree only to use 'psychological techniques of induction' in order to avoid prosecution for assault—but there are still no regulations restricting those who are not members.

Another way in which a hypnotist might cause physical damage to his subjects was demonstrated in a show which was reported on in the magazine *Picture Post* in 1952. Peter Casson (1921-1995) was, at that time, a very popular hypnotist who was attracting large audiences all round the UK and elsewhere. On this particular occasion, one of his subjects was "tiny eighteen year old Marina Gulley" who "had one chair put under her head and another under her heels, and her body was rendered so stiff by hypnosis that she could carry two twelve stone men on her unsupported middle."

Although hypnotists who used this trick maintained that subjects suffered no ill effects afterwards, the renowned American psychiatrist and hypnotherapist Milton Erickson recorded over a dozen cases of unexplained back problems in people who had been treated in the same way as Marina during a hypnosis show.

Nowadays, these physical tricks are used far less frequently. But, as we have seen, inappropriate suggestions can cause harm as well. In his classic work *Medical and Dental Hypnosis*, hypnotherapist John Hartland wrote about after-effects ranging from panic attacks through to psychosis or even suicide.

In an adjournment debate in the House of Commons in December 1994, Colin Pickthall, the Member of Parliament for Lancashire West, expressed his concerns about stage hypnosis:

> "I have had letters from all over the country giving disturbing accounts of the effects of stage hypnosis . . . Mr. Cannon from Barnet in the summer of 1992 was hypnotized and as a result he has had violent headaches ever since. He describes it as having made his life hell. Mr. Hill of Rotherham was hypnotized . . . and is subject to violent headaches, violent uncontrollable anger and persistent panic attacks. He was hospitalized several times on antidepressants and has a permanent sleeping disorder.
>
> "Dean Chambers from Blackpool had his arm paralysed for four weeks as a result of the condition

under which he was placed under hypnosis. A young man from High Wycombe [Christopher Gates] had to go to a psychiatric unit two days later where he was detained for six weeks and was still receiving treatment seven weeks later. While he was hypnotised he was put into regression, which is against the code of conduct, and was left unattended, which is also against the guidelines.

"Mr. Nickson of Prestatyn became unable to work as a result of stage hypnotism, and was unable to hold a conversation and has attempted suicide. His case is attested by Mr. Trevelyn, the consultant psychiatrist for Clwyd. David Burill of Blackpool was hypnotized . . . and collapsed immediately after being brought round. He went crazy—his words—and had to be rehypnotized. He suffered from violent headaches for weeks afterwards.

"Ruth McLoughlin, a Glasgow University student, was hypnotized in October . . . and doctors found afterwards that her heart rate had dropped to a dangerously low level.

"Dr. Prem Meisra, who works in Glasgow, described a patient who became a compulsive eater of onions after being told to eat onions instead of apples while in a trance. It sounds funny but it is not. Another of his patients went into a trance again every time someone clapped, and a further patient began to suffer from a schizoaffective disorder."

102

The British Medical Association, too, was aware of a number of cases where stage hypnosis had produced worrying or alarming results. One young man had been told, while in trance, that when he awoke he would be "on top of the world". This was another case of the subject's subconscious mind taking an instruction literally—after the performance he climbed onto a 100 foot high parapet and had to be rescued by firemen.

One of the main criticisms that medical hypnotherapists have of stage hypnotists is that they have no knowledge whatsoever of their subjects. One well known British hypnotist has been recorded as saying, when asking for volunteers "If you are drunk, mental or pregnant, don't volunteer for the show." All very well—but how many drunk people will acknowledge that they are drunk? And how many people with a mental problem will be aware of that, let alone admit to it?

Fortunately, considering the number of people who have taken part in stage hypnosis shows, the number of unpleasant side effects is probably relatively low. But the danger is ever-present. In the *Picture Post* article about Peter Casson's performance, the reporter wrote:

> "Before waking up his subjects for the interval, Casson warned them: "Whenever this tune is played in the theatre this evening you will go very deeply to sleep" . . . One girl returning . . . from the bar while the tune was being played became a dead-weight in her boyfriend's arms as she walked down the gangway.

"The hypnotist fed his guests on imaginary chickens, convinced all of them that they were full to bursting, one of them that he had indigestion . . . Casson got [the volunteers] tipsy on water, telling them all that it was rum. At one point, when the victims were standing in a somnambulant row, one massively built character fell sideways. The people all the way down the line tottered and fell, like ninepins, one by one.

"Darts experts found that, under Casson's influence, they couldn't hit the board at three feet; or more distressing, that they couldn't let go of the darts. The most hilarious moment was when the boys and girls, arbitrarily paired, kissed each other goodnight with abandon."

There was opportunity here for physical injury. If the girl who suddenly became a dead weight had not been with someone who could catch her, she could have hurt herself as she went down. Similarly, when the 'massively built character' fell and knocked the others over, someone could easily have sustained an injury. And if someone with a digestive problem, such as a peptic ulcer, had been made to experience indigestion, it could have precipitated pain that would continue once the trance had been lifted.

Perhaps one of the most worrying suggestions was that the volunteers were given water and told that it was rum. Lord Brain (1895-1996), an eminent neurologist and President of the Royal College of Physicians, wrote in a letter to the Times in 1951 that "it is not certain that hypnotism cannot be used to reinforce impulses which the subject in his conscious state is striving to suppress". In other words, a recovering alcoholic who was told under hypnosis that he was drinking rum and getting drunk might find it hard to get back on the wagon afterwards.

One thing that most hypnotherapists will do during a session is ego-strengthening—giving their patients suggestions which will increase their self-confidence and feeling of self worth. The suggestions given to the darts players were the complete opposite of this. Suddenly to find that you can't do something that you believed you were good at can be very demoralizing and the self-doubt engendered could linger on long after the subject has come out of hypnosis.

As to the kissing . . . there is no guarantee that every subject was unattached. It is not beyond the realms of possibility that seeing a boyfriend, girlfriend, husband or wife passionately kissing someone else could have caused further problems in a relationship that was already shaky.

In his speech to the House of Commons, having spoken of what he saw as the dangers of stage hypnosis, Colin Pickthall went on to say "I have not come here tonight to urge a ban on stage hypnotism . . . although my instinct is that a ban is needed". He then went on to describe what he saw as three different groups who used hypnosis:

"First, there are the legitimate and trained professional users of hypnosis for medical reasons . . . Secondly, there are the societies of stage hypnotists [who] seek codes of conduct and licensing regulations that will protect the reputation of what they view as responsible stage hypnotism . . . Thirdly, there are the unorganised, individual pirates, many of whom seem not to care in the least about the after-effects of what they do . . . We would not entertain for a moment the idea of untrained, unskilled, unlicensed people operating on people's bodies . . . but we seem to be prepared to allow untrained, unlicensed people to operate in people's minds."

CHAPTER SIX: REGRESSION

Perhaps the technique that causes the most disagreement among hypnotherapists themselves is that of regression. Some are vigorously in favor of its use, while others are just as vigorously against it. Some are happy to use 'age regression' in which patients are taken back to earlier periods in their lives, while others will go further and regress patients to the time when they were fetuses, lying in their mothers' wombs.

Still others, probably the minority, do 'past life regression' in which patients are taken back in time and are encouraged to relive events that supposedly happened to them in previous lifetimes. People who do not believe in reincarnation will, of course, dismiss past life regression as a nonsense and the stories that the patients tell while in hypnosis as pure fabrication, based on things that they have seen and read.

It is, of course, possible to fabricate under hypnosis. The visualizations in which patients see themselves coping calmly with things that have frightened them in the past are all a form of make-believe. So too are the techniques used to deepen the hypnotic trance, although these are not true fabrications since, once out of the trance, patients are aware that they were not really wandering in a garden or going down in a lift. But the whole object of the ego-strengthening type of visualization is to persuade the patient's subconscious mind that what is being imagined (for example, standing up to give a talk without one's knees knocking) is real.

The fact that hypnotized subjects seem able to remember things about their childhood which have long been forgotten, or even repressed, suggests that the memory can be greatly improved while in hypnosis. However, Professor Martin Orne, past President of the International Society of Hypnosis, once observed in a lecture that it seemed very strange that the Almighty should provide each of us with a sort of mental tape recorder which recorded all the events of our lives but which could only be turned on by a hypnotist! Actually, it is not just hypnosis that has this effect. It is not uncommon for people who are undergoing a course of psychotherapy to start remembering long-forgotten events, particularly those that have a bearing on their current problems. But, in fact, Professor Orne did demonstrate in a number of experiments that the 'memories' patients come up with, even of recent events, can be quite far from the actual truth.

Hypnosis has been used quite widely in the United States to assist in the interrogation of witnesses to crimes, in an attempt to enable them to recall more about the event than they otherwise might. However, the increasing awareness that such memories might be false and the fact that it is possible for memories to be manipulated under hypnosis means that the circumstances in which such evidence can be acquired is now strictly regulated and, in some states, it is no longer admissible.

A number of investigators have run experiments to try to see what the exact effect of hypnosis is upon a witness. Most have demonstrated that those witnesses who have recalled additional information while under hypnosis are likely, afterwards, to be very certain of the truth of what they have remembered. So it seems that one of the effects of hypnosis can be to persuade subjects that their memories are accurate—even if they're not!

In addition, it is perfectly possible for subjects knowingly to tell lies under hypnosis, so the fact that information has been given while in a trance is not even a guarantee that the subjects themselves believed this information to be true. And several investigators have noted the tendency of witnesses to confabulate while in hypnosis—in other words, if they come to a gap in their memory, they unconsciously make something up to fill it—and then later come to believe that this made-up information is true.

Professor Martin Orne did a great deal of work on forensic hypnosis (the use of hypnosis in criminal cases) and showed that it was perfectly possible to put something into the mind of hypnotized subjects which they would later state to be the truth. And this needn't be the result of an unscrupulous hypnotist 'nobbling' the witnesses—it could be done in all innocence, simply by using a phrase or sentence that might suggest something to the patient's subconscious mind.

In the 1980s, the BBC showed a program on hypnosis in which Professor Orne hypnotized a subject who had said, before the session, that on a certain night during the week she had slept soundly and had not woken once. He showed how very easy it was to use what, in legal terms, might be called leading questions to persuade the subject that she had, in fact, been woken up during that night by a loud noise in the street outside. The experiment was so successful that when the subject awoke from hypnosis she was firmly convinced not only that she had been woken by a loud noise on that particular night but also that it had taken her some time to get to sleep again.

However, although it is possible to demonstrate that such 'memories' can be fabricated, it does not necessarily mean that all memories produced under hypnosis are false. In fact, most of us will have experienced a hypnosis-like state helping to jog our memories. We have probably all, at some time, forgotten a name or an important fact—something we couldn't look up and that kept nagging at us during the course of the day, without anything coming to mind. And then, once we'd gone to bed, just as we were dropping off to sleep, we suddenly opened our eyes and said the name or fact that had eluded us all day. The state between sleeping and waking, although fairly fleeting, is very similar to a hypnotic trance and it is as we drift into this state of relaxation that the memory that we are seeking comes rushing back.

AGE REGRESSION

There are certainly cases of people being put into hypnosis and remembering things far back in their childhood with an accuracy which is later confirmed by parents or other members of the family. There are also cases of people 'remembering' events that apparently never happened to them. So does it matter whether the event is real or imagined? If one is talking in terms of hypnotherapy and not the forensic use of hypnosis, the answer is probably no.

The object of regression therapy is to bring something out from the patient's subconscious mind which is troubling him, so that it can be worked with and resolved.

For example, a patient may suffer from claustrophobia as a result of having been accidentally locked in a cupboard when he was three years old. His conscious mind has probably long since forgotten the incident, knowing that the episode happened a long time ago and is no longer relevant to his life. But the emotions associated with the experience are still active in his subconscious mind and, whenever he is in a confined space, he is subconsciously reminded of the emotions evoked by being shut in a cupboard. As a result he starts to feel apprehension and fear.

If the original event that caused the present symptoms was particularly traumatic, then it is possible for the conscious mind to blot it out completely. But it is not possible for the subconscious mind to blot out the associated emotions, and it is from these that the problem stems.

To bring out into the open the events that precipitated conditions such as claustrophobia may help the patient considerably in dealing with the problem. Many of us have experienced that feeling of being anxious but not knowing what is causing the anxiety. Then, suddenly, we become aware of what it is that is nagging and, with that realization, the anxiety becomes greatly reduced as it falls into perspective. The very fact of not knowing the cause was, in itself, contributing to the anxiety. Similarly, anxiety or emotions related to past events that we do not remember are very often out of all perspective to the causative event. For the patient to be able to remember and talk about the cause and see it from the perspective of life as it is now can be a major step towards recovery.

But what of 'memories' brought up by the patient under hypnosis that appear to have no basis in truth? Can they be of any value? Here again, the answer seems to be yes. There are many cases in which patients have been helped by visualizing and talking about some traumatic event which appears never to have happened.

Remembering a genuine past event can allay the anxiety associated with it by focusing the attention on the cause of that anxiety. But an apparently imagined focus appears to act in the same way. In other words, it seems not to matter whether the 'memory' is genuine or imagined, because in either case it seems to bring something out of the patient's subconscious mind which either is, or symbolizes, the cause of the anxieties and can therefore act to bring these anxieties into perspective.

PRIMAL THERAPY AND HYPNOSIS

Between the two areas of regression to a younger age and regression to a past life lies regression to the time when we were in our mothers' wombs and the process of being born. One might wonder why regression to this period should have any relevance to a patient's problems but, according to practitioners of 'primal therapy', the brainchild of American psychologist Dr. Arthur Janov, the events occurring before, during and after birth can, if traumatic, affect our emotional state for the rest of our lives.

112

The basic theory behind primal therapy is that unmet needs occurring early in life cause physical or psychological pain. If the pain is very severe and if, because of its severity, it is suppressed, it cannot be released from the system. Suppressed pain may be converted into tension and this, in turn, may produce other symptoms. However, if patients switch off their awareness of the tension or of the pain, psychotic mental states may occur in which they lose touch with reality.

Patients who are suffering from neuroses unconsciously use tension as a protective mechanism because, if they allowed themselves to relax, they would be able to feel the pain which their bodies and minds are suppressing. Primal therapy allows patients to feel and deal with the pain from which they are suffering, and thus relieve their neuroses.

Birth is a fairly traumatic business and, if the primal therapists are to be believed, it is small wonder that so many people have difficulty in coping with life without anxiety and tension. Ideally, a child should be wanted from the start, delivered normally and easily, and held and loved by its mother from the moment the cord is cut. However, often this is not possible. Despite modern obstetric methods, some births are still difficult and a certain number of deliveries entail the use of forceps or a Cesarean section. And sometimes, even with a normal delivery, babies have to be whisked away from their mothers immediately after birth, either because they are premature or sickly or because their mothers are unwell.

If a pregnant woman has an inadequate dietary intake or smokes or drinks heavily, her child will be unable to grow properly in the womb and is going to have unmet needs which, in primal terms, equal pain. Birth itself is bound to cause pain, say the primal therapists, because after nine months of comfort and warmth and safety in the womb, suddenly the child is being turned out to face something quite unknown. The passage down the birth canal can be very frightening and, if it takes a long time, may cause claustrophobia in later life.

If there are difficulties with the delivery because the baby has the umbilical cord around its neck, this too may be associated with difficulties later in life, such as anorexia, speech problems or problems with breathing (such as asthma). And if the child, having gone through all this trauma, does not have the immediate comfort and warmth of the mother's love and is not able to suckle, other problems may develop owing to the tension created by unmet needs.

It can be seen, therefore, that in the treatment of patients whose problems date back to traumas experienced around the time of birth, regression under hypnosis may be extremely useful. The technique is to allow the patients to relive and experience fully the pain that was felt at the time, in order to get it out of their system and to enable them to see that it is no longer relevant to their lives today.

PAST LIFE REGRESSION

Many phobias seem to have originated with a traumatic event. Sometimes this will be remembered consciously — for example, someone with a fear of dogs may remember being frightened by a dog when he was a small child. In this case, there's no need to get the patient to remember the incident—he already does. What is important is to help him to recognize the inappropriateness of the emotions to his present state. At the age of four or five a dog may seem enormous, whereas to an adult it is just a small animal. And it is possible to accomplish this change of thinking by giving suggestions under hypnosis.

Very often, the therapist may ask the patient to go back in his mind to the incident (or one of the incidents) which precipitated the present problem. The patient may start to describe an incident in his childhood or around the time of his birth or he may, as psychologist Dr. Edith Fiore discovered, start to describe a 'past life'. Dr. Fiore writes in her book *You Have Been Here Before* (National Guild of Hypnotists, 2005) that she is neither a believer nor a non-believer in reincarnation. However, one day a young man with severe sexual problems came to see her. She was experienced in treating patients using age regression under hypnosis and, once she had put him into a trance, she asked him to go back to the origin of his problems. His reply was "Two or three lifetimes ago, I was a Catholic priest".

Dr. Fiore believed that the patient's colourful and emotional description of life as a seventeenth century Italian priest was a fantasy. However, the next time the patient came to see her, his sexual problems had resolved. As a result, she started to use past life regression with other patients, often with extremely good results. As she says in her book, whether the images and stories that are conjured up are reality or fantasy doesn't actually matter—as long as the therapy gets results.

Of course, past life regression is not always done with therapy in mind. Sometimes it is carried out as an experiment to see whether or not reincarnation can be 'proved'. An early case of supposed past life regression, that of 'Bridey Murphy', caused quite a sensation in the mid-1950s and a book, *The Search for Bridey Murphy* by Morey Bernstein, was published by Hutchinson in 1956.

The subject had apparently regressed to the nineteenth century and taken on the persona of a young Irish girl. However, after the initial amazement this engendered, further research into the subject's background suggested that she knew—or had known in the past—a considerable amount about the time and places she described. It was therefore quite possible that the 'regression' was actually a fabrication based on her knowledge. It is only when it seems impossible that subjects could have known the facts that they produce during regression, and when these facts are verifiable, that one can hypothesize that the case may truly be one of past life regression.

My interest in this aspect of hypnosis began a number of years ago when I heard a recording made by a hypnotist in which he regressed a young woman back to the reign of George III. In this regression she became a young man—a gipsy—and spoke with a smattering of Romany words. She was able to give her name and she described how she and her cousin were in a town where a fair was being held. When a storm began, the two men took shelter in a barn which was then struck by lightning, and both were killed. The young woman, said the hypnotist, had never been to this town.

116

However, when taken there after she had described it in her regression, she recognized the older parts—and found a tombstone with the gipsy's name on it in the graveyard. Of course, it is impossible to say whether or not she had really ever been there—we can't remember every single place that we have ever visited. And I am unsure whether the 'Romany' she spoke was ever verified—although, certainly, the one word I remember her using ('hotchi' meaning 'hedgehog') appears in George Borrow's *Romano Lavolil: Wordbook of the Romany*, published in 1874.

The first introduction that many people in the UK had to the idea of past life regression was in 1976, through the television program *The Bloxham Tapes* and its accompanying book *More Lives Than One?* (Pan, 1976). In these, television producer Jeffrey Iverson investigated the work of Arnall Bloxham, President of the British Society of Hypnotherapists, who had been practicing past life regression for some twenty years and had recorded sessions with over 400 subjects.

Iverson began his research by listening to these recordings, but he also wanted to watch Bloxham in action. A colleague volunteered to be a subject and Bloxham regressed her to a life in ancient Greece—a period in which, so she said, she had no interest whatsoever. Iverson was impressed not only because this woman swore that she had no previous knowledge of the period but also because it was clear that Bloxham did not direct the regression in any way and asked no leading questions.

As far as the recordings were concerned, Iverson was surprised to find that most of the hypnotized subjects told stories of very ordinary, boring lives. As he wrote in the book, "If what the psychiatrists said was true, and people were fantasizing about themselves, then most were pitching their fantasies modestly and surprisingly low". But there were a few subjects who stood out, and Iverson arranged to meet them. One of these, referred to in the book as 'Jane', was invited to undergo further sessions which were filmed for the program.

In all, Jane regressed to six different 'lives', three of which seemed particularly interesting. In the first she was Livonia, the wife of a tutor of Latin and Greek, living on the outskirts of York in the third century. Some years after the program was broadcast, this particular regression was shown up as likely to be a fabrication by journalist and ardent 'debunker' Melvin Harris. Harris maintained that subjects didn't need to have a knowledge of a particular period in order to make up a story about it, because their 'facts' may well have been gleaned from historical fiction. In this particular case, he pointed out that Louis de Wohl had written a novel called *The Living Wood* (published in 1947) whose storyline had strong similarities to the story of 'Livonia', with even the names of some of the characters being the same.

Another 'life' to which Jane regressed was that of a Jewish woman named Rebecca who lived in York in the late twelfth century and who was killed in the uprising against the Jews in the city in 1189. In this regression, she came up with a large number of facts that were verified by Professor Barrie

Dobson, from the department of medieval history at York University. A number of these facts were not readily available in books, suggesting that Jane could not have remembered them from her reading. In addition, there seemed to be no work of fiction which in any way related to her story.

But the most impressive regression was perhaps the one in which Jane found herself as Alison, a servant girl to a nobleman, Jacques Coeur, in the Loire Valley in the mid-fifteenth century. Jane said that she had never been to the Loire Valley nor studied its history—facts that were easily verified by Iverson who happened to have gone to the same school and knew the history syllabus. And yet she was able to describe the house in which she had lived as a servant (which still stands) and to talk, correctly, about the relationships of various people at Court.

She also spoke about her master's collection of art, including paintings by Fouquet, van Eyck and John of Bruges. Both Fouquet and van Eyck were court painters, so it would have been possible for her to know their names, but John of Bruges was more obscure and his name appears only in specialist textbooks.

But one item in Coeur's collection was harder to trace. She described it as a 'golden apple' which he had prized highly. After much research, a local historian, searching through archives of the period, found a list of 'items confiscated by the Treasury from Jacques Coeur' when he was arrested on a trumped up charge of murder. And in that list was a 'grenade [or pomegranate] of gold'—in other words, an item that looked very much like an apple.

Melvin Harris, having cast doubt on the regression to 'Livonia' tried again with 'Alison'. But this time his case was very unconvincing. He cited a novel by Thomas Costain, called *The Moneyman* which was published in 1947 and republished in 1961 and had Jacques Coeur as its central character. But the majority of characters in the novel are fictional, as is the story which does not relate in any way to Alison's life. Indeed, many of the facts that Jane came up with were quite obscure and were not in any of the readily available history books.

Nearly ten years after *The Bloxham Tapes* was aired, another program on reincarnation was shown on British television—this time on Channel 4. It followed the course of an experiment carried out by Australian psychologist and hypnotherapist, Peter Ramster, who was an experienced past-life regressionist. Out of the many subjects he had regressed, he picked four women who not only produced vivid and detailed descriptions of their past lives but, in addition, had never visited the countries in which they had seen themselves living (England, Scotland, France and Germany). Indeed, one of them had never been out of Australia.

All the regression was done in Australia and as much information as possible was requested from the subjects and recorded. Then the four women were taken to Europe, to the places to which they had apparently regressed, and were asked to find their way around.

One of the four, who had described life as a Jewish girl in Nazi Germany, found that the streets were not as she had described them, nor were buildings in the places that she had said they were. It seems likely, therefore, that in her case the vivid imagery was based on something that she had read or seen on television. Since there is so much material available on Nazi Germany, this is totally plausible.

However, the woman who described her life in a grand house in France was able to take Peter Ramster on a guided tour of that house (now derelict). She also described (accurately, as it turned out) a house, several miles away, at which she had spent a number of summers and, without looking at a map, was able to give directions which took them from one house to the other.

The woman who had regressed to a small English village in the eighteenth century talked, while in hypnosis, about a friend of hers whose cottage had a strange pattern carved in the stone floor. Before leaving Australia, she was asked to draw that pattern. When she arrived in the village, the cottage was still standing, although it had for many years been used as a hen-house. But when the hens were turned out and the floor cleaned, the pattern she had drawn was discovered there.

Equally amazing was the woman who had described her life as a doctor in a Scottish town. She was able to point out where the Seamen's Mission had stood in the early nineteenth century (a fact unknown to local historians, who were only able to confirm it after delving into records). And finding, without difficulty, the building which had once been the medical school, she correctly identified the use to which several of the rooms had been put at that period — and where the gentlemen's toilet had been. A map from the university archives confirmed these facts as true — but the map had apparently never been reproduced.

Although such results are greeted with delight by those who believe in reincarnation, there are, of course, people who feel that there must be some other explanation. Perhaps one of the commonest criticisms made is that a subject, while accurate in some respects, hasn't got everything right. But here we have to remember the fact, noted earlier in this chapter, that people in trance tend to fill gaps in their memories by making something up. It is therefore quite possible, if one allows for the reality of reincarnation, for someone under hypnosis to remember part of a past life and fill in the gaps with something he has imagined.

Another argument. frequently put forward by those who believe that all past life regressions are imaginary, concerns language. If someone spoke Romany, or French, or Italian, or ancient Egyptian in a previous life and if, in hypnosis, they appear to be reliving their experiences in that life, then one would expect them to recount those experiences in the language that they spoke at the time. This would seem to be a very sound argument. Some subjects, of course, do speak partly in their 'previous' language (such as the 'gipsy' with his smattering of Romany) and partly in their present-day language. Others will speak only in their present language but will offer words in their previous tongue if requested.

Some appear unable to recall any of their previous language, although remembering quite a lot about the relevant lifetime.

One way in which such phenomena may be explained is this: it is rather like the situation of someone who, as a small child, was brought up in a household in which French was spoken fluently. At the age of five, he was taken away and put in another household where only English was spoken, and he never spoke French again. At the age of 65 he is asked, in English, about his life as a small child. He may be able to remember certain events quite vividly, but he will describe them in English. However, if there were certain words or phrases that made a particular impression on him (perhaps a term of endearment used towards him) he is likely to repeat that in the original French. When pressed, he may even be able to remember some other French words that have remained dormant in his mind for 60 years.

Similarly, when people describe, in hypnosis, what it was like to be born, they do so in adult terms, although obviously they knew no language at the time. Some years ago I was treating a patient with hypnosis and asked him to go back in time to the first incident which had contributed to his present problems. Knowing something of the patient's childhood, I expected this to be an event when he was about four or five years old. I was therefore somewhat surprised when he said "I'm lying near a naked woman". He paused and then said "There are other people about. And I've got a rushing noise in my ears. There's a strong artificial light and I can hear bells. I'm hot and I feel tingling and unpleasant. I feel as though I'm floating—it seems as though I'm being lifted up. And now I'm shouting. I feel very frustrated—I want something but I don't know what it is." He was, of course, describing events shortly after he had been born. And although, as a newborn baby, he could only express his frustration by crying (or 'shouting'), he was now describing it in the language of a 30 year old man.

TECHNIQUES FOR REGRESSION

There are many methods used by hypnotherapists to help subjects to regress. The simplest is that used by Arnall Bloxham in which the subject is just asked to go back in time. Dr. Edith Fiore's method is to suggest to the subject that he travel back through time and space while she counts slowly to ten; when she reaches ten, while still being himself, the subject will find that he is in another time and another place and another body, but all of these will be relevant to his present problems. A method which is useful when the subject is being regressed just a short way, perhaps a matter of a few years, is to ask him to imagine a calendar and to see it going backwards until the required date is reached.

Subjects need to be able to go into a medium-depth or deep trance in order to be regressed and, even then, there may be resistance, particularly if they have been suppressing painful memories for years. However, there are ways to get round this. One is for the therapist to say "I'm going to count to five, and while I'm counting something will come into your mind that will give us a clue as to the cause of your current problems". This 'something' may be something the subject sees (such as a scene or a face), or a non-visual clue such as a noise or a snatch of tune, a smell or even an emotion.

124

The subject is told to allow his mind to go completely blank and just allow whatever it is to come into his mind. It may appear to have no relevance to the problem, so he is not to discard any thought or emotion that suddenly appears, no matter how trivial it may seem. This technique needs a reasonable depth of trance because it is important that the conscious mind is overridden by the subconscious. A patient whose trance is too light will either come up with what he consciously thinks is relevant or will come up with nothing, saying something along the lines of "I'm sorry, I can't think of anything that might have caused it".

A similar method is to ask the hypnotized subject to give three letters of the alphabet off the top of his head. Then he is asked, again without thinking about it, to say three words, each beginning with one of the letters, and each of which will be relevant to his problem. And finally, he is asked to put each of the words into a sentence. With both this method and the previous one, what has come into the subject's mind or the sentences he produces have then to be developed and enlarged upon. Of course, using these particular methods, the subject may not regress, since there may be things in his life as it is at present that are of great relevance to his problems, and it may be these that come to mind.

Quite often patients are nervous that there may be something traumatic in their past which they are going to be required to remember. However, although it is often important to re-experience the emotions associated with traumatic events, in order to get them out of the system, the edge can be taken off by suggestions from the therapist that the patient will remain calm and relaxed throughout the session. Because patients can be aware of being both in a different time and in the hypnotherapist's chair, it is possible to experience emotion generated by the regression while at the same time remaining relaxed in the present. Perhaps the closest analogy to this is watching a 'weepy' film on television. While dabbing your eyes with a tissue because of the moving events on the screen, you are still very much aware that you are sitting in a comfortable chair in your own home and that the emotion you are feeling is relevant only to that film and not to your life.

The image of a television set or a cinema screen can, in fact, be used to protect patients from events that are very traumatic. Instead of being asked to go back and experience such events, they can be asked to imagine that they are watching a film of them. They will be aware of the emotions that the people on the screen are going through because they are those people but, because they are detached from the scene, they will not be unduly upset by them.

After revisiting a trauma, it is often helpful to take patients forward to some time after the event, to a more peaceful episode, to show them that they survived the trauma and so give them confidence in their own strength and resilience. Even with patients who see themselves dying in former lives, continuing on after the death will often produce a profound sense of peace and, if they then move forward into the current life, it will show them that everything can be overcome.

In *More Lives Than One?* Jeffrey Iverson describes a patient of Arnall Bloxham's who was afraid of going to sleep in case he

126

should die. Bloxham's solution was to regress the patient to previous lives in order to convince him that he had lived — and, more to the point, died — many times before and that, as a result, death should hold no surprises or terrors for him.

Another method in which a sense of detachment from traumatic events can be created is the visualization of a 'Book of Life'. This technique can be extremely useful to help a patient explore his current life from an early age. He is asked to imagine a bookshelf on which there are several books labelled 'My Life: Volume 1', 'My Life: Volume 2' and so on, the number of volumes depending on the age of the individual patient. At the first session, he is asked to picture himself taking the first book off the shelf, then sitting down and opening it. Each page is like a television screen with a moving picture showing an event that is of significance.

Volume One will start with events when the patient was very young (perhaps up to the age of five and the first day at school). He is asked to look at each picture in turn and to describe what is happening and how he feels about it. When he has talked at length about each picture and the emotions with which he associates it, he is given a choice. If he considers that the memories that the page conjured up were happy ones and he wants to keep them, then all he has to do is to turn the page over and go on to the next. If, however, the memories are unhappy or traumatic ones, he can tear the page out, screw it up and throw it away — and it will not trouble him again. This is a particularly useful method when a series of minor events has contributed to a patient's problems, but less so when one or more very traumatic episodes are involved.

Obviously it is important that sessions of regression should not be traumatic for the patient. Long-standing problems may take a number of sessions of hypnotherapy before they start to resolve and, if the patient is going to be too scared to return for another session, then the technique is pointless. On some occasions, therefore, it may be necessary for a patient to be allowed to forget what has happened under hypnosis, while his subconscious mind works it out. Many hypnotherapists will routinely tell patients that, when they wake up, they will remember only the parts of the session with which the conscious mind is able to cope. Patients then have the choice as to what they remember and what they forget.

CHAPTER SEVEN: SOME COMMON CONDITIONS & THEIR TREATMENT

In this chapter, we shall look at how a medical hypnotherapist might treat various conditions. It is important to remember, however, that new treatment techniques are being developed all the time and many more exist than can be described in a single chapter. So if you go to see a hypnotherapist you will not necessarily encounter any of the methods mentioned here. Naturally, therapists use the techniques that seem to them to give the best results, and the fact that two practitioners may use quite different methods doesn't necessarily mean that one is more skilled, or even more up to date, than the other. However, it may mean that sometimes a patient will get on better with one therapist than with another. This is something that hypnotherapists recognize and this is the reason why, very occasionally, a patient may be referred from one to another.

SMOKING

A large percentage of the people who seek help from hypnotherapists do so because they want to stop smoking. So if you're thinking of trying hypnotherapy to help you quit, it's quite likely that you've been spurred on by knowing someone else for whom it worked. However, as we have already noted, it can only help you if you really want to give up. If the main reasons you smoke are habit and nicotine addiction there's a very good chance that you'll be successful. However, if you're one of those people who really enjoys the taste of the cigarette and gets satisfaction from the ritual involved in smoking it might not be as easy. But even if you do fall into this second group, hypnotherapy may still be able to help you if you have a very strong reason to give up (such as anxieties about your health) because it will help to strengthen your will-power to do what you know has to be done.

Many people who smoke do so in order to relieve tension. If you're someone who needs a cigarette when you're anxious or you're working under pressure, hypnosis could really help you. Because hypnosis is, essentially, a relaxation technique, it can help to reduce your tensions so that you no longer need to smoke. When you're in trance, the therapist is likely to tell you that you're going to start feeling more relaxed in your everyday life and will find that the sort of situations that have tended to make you feel tense and anxious will no longer do so. This sense of calm will build up gradually and, as a result, you will no longer have the need to smoke that you did previously. Smoking was just a crutch—now you can keep yourself calm and relaxed without artificial aids.

People who plan to give up smoking have a choice of ways in which to do it, whatever methods or therapies they choose to help them. They can either decide that on a certain day they will stop and not start again, or they can cut down gradually until, finally, they stop. If you're intending to try hypnosis to help you quit, and you have a strong preference either for the cold turkey method or for giving up gradually, it's important to mention this to your therapist at the first session, so that the post-hypnotic suggestions that you are given will be appropriate.

One way to help you give up gradually, is to ask you to record your progress on a chart. Then, while you are in hypnosis, you may be asked to visualize the chart as it will appear in two or three weeks' time, seeing how well you are doing. You may also be asked to look ahead to see what the date will be when you finally give up. The more clearly you can see the date, the more likely it is that you will be able to stop. Patients who have difficulty seeing the date are often not very committed to cutting down and may find it easier just to stop. But if you can see the date, you may be asked to imagine the events on that day—the feeling of achievement and the delight of your family or your friends or even your doctor (whoever is currently complaining most about your smoking!).

If you are taught self-hypnosis, you will be able to use these visualizations every time you practice it and this will reinforce the work you do in the sessions with your hypnotherapist. Hopefully, your family and friends will encourage you in your efforts because it's much harder to stop if other members of your family are still puffing away. If you live with another smoker (or smokers) you may be able to arrange to be seen together by the hypnotherapist so you can work together on giving up and give each other mutual support and encouragement.

It has to be said that giving up smoking can be difficult even if you have a strong motivation and will-power to do it. Many people, whether they give up suddenly or gradually, suffer from withdrawal effects, sometimes for a considerable period of time. The various nicotine preparations available nowadays can help with this but they aren't suitable for everyone, being contraindicated, for example, in pregnancy and in people with a history of angina or heart attack. But hypnotherapy does away with the need for nicotine patches.

The commonest withdrawal effects that people complain of are craving for a cigarette, irritability, insomnia and wanting to eat all the time. These can all be treated—the irritability and insomnia can be overcome by teaching you how to relax and how to use self-hypnosis to get yourself to sleep at night. Your therapist is likely to ask you when it is that you feel the greatest need for a cigarette—for example, after a meal, when drinking a cup of coffee, or when you're on the 'phone—and will then give you specific suggestions that you will not feel a need to smoke at these times or, of course, at any other.

You may be given a special technique to use at difficult times—for example, you may be told that, when the craving starts, if you snap your fingers it will immediately disappear and be replaced by a sensation of relaxation and well-being. And, if eating more is likely to be a problem, you may be told that, while it is likely that you will enjoy your food more as a result of being able to taste it better, you will have no desire to eat more than you usually do.

It's possible that you're one of those people who find you can do without cigarettes quite happily until you get into an environment where other people are smoking. Then, if you're offered a cigarette, the smell of the smoke makes it very hard to resist. This, too, can be overcome because your hypnotherapist can give you a suggestion that not only will the smell of smoke not encourage you to smoke, but you will find the smell of other people smoking very unpleasant. And you'll start to wonder why you ever smoked. You may also be told that, if you do succumb and light a cigarette, it will taste vile and you won't be able to put it out quickly enough! This can be a very effective suggestion and some of my patients have reported a dramatic change in the perceived flavour of tobacco.

Suggestions such as these, which depend on patients experiencing something which is not so, may be more easily accepted by the subconscious mind if they are coupled with suggestions that are based on reality. So, for example, you may be told that when you stop smoking you will find that your food tastes much better and you'll be far more aware of pleasant smells in your environment. This, of course, will happen anyway as your senses of taste and smell, which have been suppressed by smoking, start to return to normal. But the very fact that it does happen, just as you were told when you were in a trance, will encourage your subconscious mind to believe everything else that you've been told under hypnosis. So you may be told that it is because of your improved sense of taste that any cigarette you light will taste so bad.

You may also be given 'automatic reaction' suggestions such as "If someone offers you a cigarette, you will automatically say 'No thank you, I've given up'". For people who are good subjects and well motivated, this can be a very effective technique because the reaction will occur without them even thinking about it and will therefore help them to avoid being tempted to have 'just one'. The technique is, in fact, exactly the same one that is used by stage hypnotists to make a subject do or say something on a given signal once they're out of trance and back in the audience. What is a source of amusement in the hands of a stage hypnotist may be a very valuable therapeutic tool in the hands of a hypnotherapist.

Self hypnosis is very important if you want to give up smoking. Patients who practice it regularly seem to do much better than those who don't. It may be, of course, that those who practice more do so because they're determined to succeed, but there is no doubt that their task is made easier by their increased ability to relax, greater self-reliance and improved confidence in their own ability to stop smoking— all of which are results of regular practice.

My own experience with treating smokers suggests that the best self-hypnosis schedule is 20 minutes a day while you're in the process of giving up, and until you feel confident that you're unlikely to relapse, and then 20 minutes two or three times a week—probably for the rest of your life. In this way, if you ever find yourself open to the temptation to start again, you'll have the techniques at hand to help you to resist.

Response to treatment varies considerably from patient to patient. Some find no difficulty at all in stopping smoking or in cutting down and then stopping. Others take longer than they intended, but give up eventually. Others seem to get nowhere. For those patients who have made no progress after three sessions of hypnosis, the likelihood that it's going to help is small, and they would probably be best advised to try another method (such as an acupuncture stud) or to return to hypnosis at a later date when they are feeling more committed to quitting.

Occasionally, someone who has given up smoking with the aid of hypnotherapy, will start again. So a therapist may see people who quit several years earlier coming back, rather shame-faced, for a repeat performance. Usually they have let their practice of self-hypnosis lapse and, often, they are worried as to whether the therapy will work a second time. In most cases it does, although sometimes it may be harder to give up than on the previous occasion, since the patient's self-confidence has taken a knock. However, as with first-time patients, it is the motivation that is important, and those who really want to give up will do so.

INSOMNIA

Insomnia is a very common problem and can often be caused by conditions such as anxiety or pain. However, it may also occur by itself, for no apparent reason, and it is in these cases that hypnotherapy may prove useful. Of course, it is also a valuable treatment for anxiety and pain (see later sections in this chapter) but, in such a case, it would be the underlying condition that required treatment rather than the insomnia.

Because the identification of underlying conditions is so important, the therapist is likely to take a full history of the problem so that the treatment given is appropriate. It may appear to the patient that there is no reason for his disturbed sleep, but a medical hypnotherapist may be able to see a very obvious reason. For example, there are some people who don't allow anything to worry them. No matter what happens, they continue to show a cheerful face and carry on regardless. It's not that things *don't* worry them, it's just that

135

they suppress such things and refuse to acknowledge them. They may not even be aware that they are doing this or, if they are, may be very reluctant to admit it.

There are many people, mainly women, who spend their lives looking after an elderly parent or an invalid spouse and, often, such people feel guilty if they allow worry, anxiety or fatigue to show. But emotions have to have an outlet; if a natural outlet is denied them, the emotions will express themselves in another way and cause psychosomatic disease. Insomnia may be an early sign of such bottled-up emotions and hypnosis can offer a gentle way of allowing the patient to release her feelings and accept them for what they are.

In such a case, the patient would be encouraged, under hypnosis, to talk about how she felt and would be allowed to express emotions such as anger and resentment that it was impossible for her to show to the person in her care. Gradually she could come to feel that expression of her emotions was not wrong but, on the contrary, was a perfectly natural reaction to circumstances. She could also be reassured that there was no disloyalty involved in her 'letting go' like this because, as a result, her relationship with the person she cared for could improve, so that they would both benefit. Finally she could learn how to recognize her emotions and to deal with them, instead of bottling them up and allowing them to cause illness.

Anxiety does not always express itself simply as an inability to sleep. Some patients suffer from recurrent nightmares.

These produce a two-fold effect: not only do they disturb the patient's sleep, but they also make him dread going back to sleep or even falling asleep in the first place. When a patient is in a hypnotic trance, these dreams can be explored. The examination of any episode or theme that seems to recur frequently may give clue as to the underlying anxiety.

If you have been suffering from nightmares, your therapist may suggest that you re-experience them while in a hypnotic trance. However, since you are consciously going to make a decision to bring these frightening scenes into your mind, you will also be able to control them. The therapist can then help you with further suggestions. For example, if you have been dreaming frequently that you are being pursued by savage dogs, your therapist may ask you to look at the animals again and see them change into something less fearsome—lambs or guineas pigs, perhaps. You may then be given a suggestion that, because the dream has now changed into something fairly innocuous, it will not recur again—or, if it does, it will be in its new form.

In addition, you may be asked to express what the dream means to you. Because the meaning is usually hidden somewhere in the subconscious mind, one of the techniques used in regression therapy may be appropriate. For example, you might be told that the symbolic meaning of a certain component of the dream will automatically come into your head when the therapist counts to five. Or you might be told that if you look really hard at whatever it is that frightens you in your dream, you will see what it really symbolizes. So, for example, if you were worried about your job and were

137

constantly being harried by your employer, the German shepherd that, in your nightmares, is forever barking and snapping at your heels might suddenly transform into an image of your boss shouting or complaining.

If the therapist tells you that something will automatically come into your mind, it is essential that you allow your mind to become blank, so that your subconscious can produce whatever image is relevant. However, many people find it difficult to do this, with the result that their answers are not spontaneous but are the result of conscious thinking. One way of getting over this problem is to use the 'ideomotor' finger signalling technique. This, in effect, allows your fingers to do the talking.

The therapist will ask you to concentrate on the word 'yes' and will tell you that, as you do so, one of your fingers will start to lift up. When this has happened, the formula is repeated with 'no', 'I don't know' and 'I don't want to tell you'. Then the therapist will tell you that he's going to ask you some questions but that you won't have to concentrate on them, or even listen to them. Your fingers will do the work for you, and you can just lie back and relax. The one drawback of this technique is that all the ideas have to come from the therapist and, although it can work well when he has a fairly clear picture of the cause of the problem, progress can be rather slow when the origins are obscure. Of course, finger signalling is not just limited to the treatment of insomnia—it can also be used in any case where it's necessary to delve into the background of the patient's complaints.

With some patients, there is no deep-seated cause for their insomnia. For them, inability to sleep is just a habit. It may have started at a time when they were anxious about something and the insomnia may have added to their anxiety. Now, with the original cause long gone, they continue to worry about their insomnia and a vicious cycle is set up whereby the anxiety produces insomnia which produces anxiety. If this vicious cycle can be broken, the patient will once again be able to sleep normally.

In cases such as this, hypnotherapy can produce dramatic results. Firstly, it can relieve patients of their anxiety by teaching them how to relax. They can be given suggestions that it doesn't really matter whether they sleep or not because, even if they don't, they won't feel exhausted. This is perfectly possible, since a lot of the exhaustion felt will be due to the anxiety and the resultant muscle tension. So, even if they are still getting fewer hours of sleep than they need, what they do get should be more restful.

In addition to breaking the vicious cycle, hypnotherapy can be used to teach patients how to get to sleep. Although hypnosis is not itself a form of sleep, it is very closely related and, in the moments before we go off to sleep, we are in a state that is very similar to a hypnotic trance. When I first started my hypnotherapy training, someone on the course asked the tutor "Is there any risk of the patient not coming out of the trance?" The tutor explained that, if this happens, it is always because the patient consciously wishes to stay in the trance. He then continued this reassurance by saying "If a patient is left in a trance, ultimately he will drift into a normal sleep from which he will wake in due course. So you mustn't worry that if you suddenly drop down dead from a heart attack something terrible will happen to your patient—he'll just go off to sleep and then wake up in due course—although not, unfortunately, in time to administer heart massage to his therapist!"

So, drifting from hypnosis into sleep is a perfectly natural phenomenon. Indeed, it is not unusual for patients who are practicing self-hypnosis to fall asleep on the odd occasion when they are feeling tired—and it's not unknown for an overtired patient to fall asleep during a session of hypnotherapy in the consulting room!

Because of this characteristic of hypnosis, if patients who are being treated for insomnia put themselves into self-hypnosis at night when they are ready to go to sleep, they will automatically drift from a hypnotic trance into a natural sleep. They may find it difficult at first but, with practice, will be able to go to sleep very quickly whenever they want to. And the two major advantages of this method, compared with the use of sleeping tablets, are that if the patient wakes in the night, the technique can be used to get back to sleep again and, of course, there will be no after-effects in the morning.

I have written extensively about the treatments that orthodox medicine and complementary therapies offer for insomnia in my book *Insomnia and Other Sleep Disorders*, published by Sphinx House.

ANXIETY

Anxiety lies at the root of many of the problems that are amenable to treatment with hypnosis. However, in many cases, it is the anxiety itself which is the main symptom. The patient will be aware of feeling anxious and tense all the time, even if she (or, less frequently, he) has nothing to be anxious about. Any upset in the daily routine, however minor, will add to the anxiety, and what might appear to the outsider to be a relatively trivial problem may seem to the patient to be insurmountable and may cause a considerable worsening of her symptoms.

Usually the patient knows that there is no real cause for her anxiety and, as a result, she worries about the way she feels which, on the one hand, seems senseless but on the other seems to be in complete control of her.

This knowledge that the way one feels or acts is irrational is commonly associated with the conditions described as neuroses in medical terminology. And, sometimes, the awareness of the irrationality of her behavior can lead the patient to believe that she must be going mad. However, patients who are suffering from the more severe mental conditions known as psychoses (and who, in the old days, would have been labelled 'mad') have no insight into their conditions and can see nothing irrational in their own behavior.

Hypnosis is only very rarely used in the treatment of psychotic patients, and then only under the supervision of a psychiatrist, since there is a possibility of it making their condition worse. Since it may sometimes be difficult to diagnose cases which lie on the borderline of psychosis, patients who want to try hypnotherapy for a purely mental condition (such as anxiety) should always consult a therapist who is either a doctor or a qualified psychologist and who will therefore be able to assess whether hypnosis is appropriate.

Some patients who are suffering from depression should also avoid hypnosis. Very often, they have, in addition to their depression, a degree of anxiety which, it might be thought, could benefit from hypnotic treatment. Unfortunately, alleviating the anxiety may make the depression worse because sometimes it is only the energy of the anxiety that is keeping the patient going.

However, for patients who are suffering solely from anxiety, without any coexistent depression, hypnotherapy can be extremely helpful. But, here again, it is advisable to consult a therapist who is also a doctor or psychologist, since the symptoms of clinical depression are quite different from the feeling of simply being depressed and it may not be easy for the patient herself to judge whether she is suffering from anxiety alone or from anxiety plus depression.

Before the advent of tranquilizers, patients who suffered from anxiety and the associated tendency to panic attacks could be severely incapacitated when it came to leading a normal life. Panic attacks can occur at any time or in any place, sometimes when the patient is away from home, perhaps out shopping or visiting friends. Because these attacks are so overwhelming, the patient may become terrified that an attack will occur when she is away from the safety of her own home, and she may therefore avoid going out as much as possible. (This is different from the condition of agoraphobia, in which the patient knows what it is that makes her anxious—that is, going out of the house—and the sensation is more one of constant overwhelming fear at all times when she is out. Panic attacks often seem to have no particular precipitating factor and may occur just as easily at home as when the patient is out.)

With the advent of tranquilizers, family doctors suddenly found that they were able to treat patients suffering from anxiety, many of whom found relief from librium, valium and similar preparations before there was any indication that such drugs could become addictive. Unfortunately, a patient who remains on tranquilizers long term may find, over time, that the tablets become less and less helpful in suppressing the symptoms, so that the dose needs to be increased. This, in turn, is likely to make the side-effects—such as lethargy and an inability to concentrate—more pronounced. And, once on tranquilizers, a patient may be very unwilling to come off them again. Even if she is aware that she feels bad while taking them, she may be scared that she will feel ten times worse after coming off.

Fortunately, hypnotherapy presents none of these problems. It has no side-effects and it doesn't become less effective over time. And, unlike tranquilizers, which merely suppress the symptoms, hypnotherapy improves the state of the patient's mind so that she is no longer anxious. As it is a self-help therapy, the patient can progress at the rate which suits her best, using regular self-hypnosis. It may even be helpful for patients who are trying to come off tranquilizers, although those who have been on them for a long time may be hard to hypnotize. (For these patients, homeopathy is probably the treatment of choice.)

Anxious patients often say that they find it impossible to relax, no matter how hard they try. Of course, the very fact that they are *trying* to do so, rather than just allowing themselves to, is probably one reason why they cannot. However, when one uses hypnosis, the word 'relaxation' need not even be mentioned. The induction and deepening of the trance may involve counting, deep breathing or a visualization and it is on these that the patient concentrates. It is therefore possible for her to relax without even being aware that she is doing so. Sometimes one can actually see the muscles and the tension lines of a patient's face relax as she sinks into a trance.

Once she is in hypnosis, the treatment of the anxious patient consists primarily in giving her confidence in her own ability to relax (which she has just demonstrated) and in teaching her how to do so. So she will often be taught self-hypnosis and will be told that, as she has now proved that she can relax while in a trance, it is just as possible for her to relax at other times. Suggestions may be given that she will start to feel very much more relaxed in her everyday life and that she will find it much easier to cope with the sorts of situations that have worried her in the past.

A patient who suffers from panic attacks may be taught specific techniques to help her to cope with them. These are really just elaborations on the 'calm and relaxed' technique mentioned in chapter four, where it is suggested that repetition of the phrase will bring about the desired effect. However, such a repetition by itself may not be enough to control an acute panic attack so she may be given something else to do as well, to reinforce the effect. One such method is for her to clench her fists and take a deep breath as soon as she feels the panic rising within her. Then she is told that she will be able to feel the panic running from her brain and from the rest of her body down her arms and into her clenched fists. Once all the panic has 'collected in her fists', she breathes out quickly and, at the same time, flings open her fists 'to throw the panic away'.

Although the patient does not have to be in a hypnotic trance when she uses this technique, it must, of course, be taught to her while she is hypnotized so that her subconscious mind will automatically do what is required when she goes through the ritual. As with most hypnotherapeutic techniques, she will probably have to practice it a number of times before it is really effective. Once it is working, however, the efficacy of the technique will be reinforced by her confidence in it and the resulting feeling of security may well prevent further attacks from occurring.

In addition to these methods of treatment, the usual ego-strengthening techniques are also used and, if there is a specific factor which is causing the patient's anxiety, this can be explored. More will be said about this in the section on the treatment of phobias.

ASTHMA

Asthma is a condition which is almost invariably associated with anxiety. In many patients the precipitating cause may be an allergic one (for example, coming into contact with pollen or cat fur) but, because being unable to breathe is so frightening, the feeling that an attack is about to start may result in a large and sudden build-up of anxiety. And this, in turn, may make what would have been a minor asthmatic attack develop into a major one. In some patients, anxiety itself can bring on an attack. And so we have a vicious cycle, with anxiety causing asthma, which causes anxiety and so on. But this means that if one can control the anxiety, one can also—to a greater or lesser extent—control the asthma.

Since asthma commonly affects children, it is fortunate that they tend to be very good subjects for hypnosis. Opinions differ as to the youngest age at which hypnosis can be used but, to a large extent, it depends on the individual child. It is important that he is old enough to concentrate on what the therapist is saying and to co-operate in the treatment. Children of six or seven usually present no problems but hypnotherapists who specialize in treating children may be happy to treat patients who are even younger than this.

When the patient is a child, the therapist, before inducing a trance, will usually start by explaining what it is that happens to the body during an asthma attack. The role of fear in the development of an attack will be stressed and the therapist will explain how it is possible to overcome the fear and so control the attack. It is important that the child should agree freely to have the treatment, otherwise it is unlikely to be beneficial. Usually a parent will be present during the treatment session. Some therapists prefer to treat children with the same condition (such as asthma or eczema) in groups rather than individually. Even when patients are hypnotized in groups, they can be treated individually since they can be told "You will remain absorbed in a pleasant daydream until I put my hand on your shoulder and call your name". So each patient will pay attention only to the suggestions that are directed specifically at him. In this way time can be saved by using one induction and deepening technique for several patients, without detracting from the quality of the treatment.

Much of the basic treatment for asthma is the same as that for anxiety. Patients, whether adults or children, are taught how to relax and how to put themselves into hypnosis. The techniques for self-hypnosis may be made simpler for children—for example, they may just be told to repeat a particular word or phrase a certain number of times. However, when teaching self-hypnosis to a child, extra precautions must be taken in addition to those normally used. For example, young patients will be told that they will only be able to put themselves into hypnosis when a parent, or other responsible adult, is in the house and knows what the child is doing. Children will also be told that they won't be able to hypnotize themselves to entertain their friends and that, if an adult calls them while they are in trance, they will immediately wake up.

As well as being taught basic relaxation techniques, asthmatic patients—whether adults or children—can be given a formula with which to break the vicious cycle of anxiety and worsening asthma. This may be something akin to the 'clenched fist' technique that was described in the section on anxiety. So they may be asked to imagine all the tension and tightness that they feel in their chest transferring to their fists, from where it can be thrown away. Or they may be given a phrase to repeat, with the suggestion that, as they do so, their breathing will become easier and their muscles will relax.

For clients who use inhalers and find them useful, a suggestion may be given along the lines of "As you repeat the phrase you have been given, you will feel just as though you have used your inhaler, knowing that the tightness is relaxing and that you are beginning to breathe normally again".

If a patient is hypnotized or uses self-hypnosis shortly after an attack has started, it will usually abate. Some therapists will, while patients are in trance, get them to feel an attack coming on, feel the tightness, feel it becoming more difficult to breathe, and then use whichever technique has been taught to relieve the attack. At first, patients may be loath to induce an attack, for fear that they will not be able to control it. However, once they have done so, it will be impressed on them that if the power of the mind is strong enough to produce an attack just by thinking about it, then it must also be strong enough to alleviate an attack. Once patients can control a self-induced attack under hypnosis, they will find it increasingly easy to control 'real' attacks.

Of course, it goes without saying that such techniques should only be taught by qualified medical hypnotherapists—that is, doctors with a training in hypnosis. Because asthma is a serious and, on occasion, life-threatening condition, it is essential that the therapist is medically trained to deal with any emergency.

There is yet another method for treating children with asthma which consists—extraordinary as it may sound—in treating their mothers. As long ago as 1941, psychoanalysts Franz Alexander and Thomas Morton French suggested that childhood asthma was a psychosomatic condition that resulted from the child's feeling of being rejected by its mother. By the 1980s this impression had been corroborated by numerous researchers. What was at fault, it seemed, was the bonding between mother and child.

Normally bonding will occur immediately after birth but there are a number of factors—both physical and emotional— that can prevent this from happening. A difficult labor, delivery by Cesarean section, or a separation of mother and baby immediately after birth may all interfere with bonding, as may postnatal depression or stress during the pregnancy (caused, for example, by marital problems or the death of a family member).

Why children who do not bond are more likely to develop asthma is unclear, although some researchers believe that it has something to do with the effect of the perceived rejection by the mother on the child's immune system. Whatever the reason, there does seem to be a clear correlation. Separate studies have shown that bonding failure is three times more likely to have happened in asthmatic children than in those who are not asthmatic.

Dr. Antonio Madrid of the University of San Francisco pioneered the use of hypnosis to treat the mothers of these children in the early 1980s and has written a number of papers on the subject. His technique has proved remarkably effective. First of all, the therapist talks to the mother about bonding, identifying the problem that interfered with this in her own case. By highlighting this, the mother can see that the failure to bond was not her fault (as she may previously have believed) and this often produces a great sense of relief.

Then the mother is hypnotized and, very simply, in her relaxed state, is told to allow all these problems to heal. She may be asked to visualize something—such as a vacuum cleaner—clearing out all the bad memories, thoughts and feelings while the subconscious mind does the healing. Once this is done, she is helped to relive her pregnancy and labor while in trance. But, this time, everything will go well and she will remain happy and relaxed throughout. Having visualized herself giving birth easily, she then sees herself holding her baby and feeling the bond growing. Of course, once she comes out of hypnosis, she will still remember what actually did happen during her pregnancy and after her child was born, but the negative emotions associated with it will have been replaced by the feelings of happiness and love created by the visualization.

This therapy is usually accomplished in four or five sessions, or less. In one study, where fifteen mothers were treated, the symptoms of twelve of the children improved and, of the ten who had been taking medication regularly, ten no longer needed it. In another study, six mothers were treated and five of the children had a total remission of all their symptoms. The children who don't respond tend to be older—the technique works best in those under the age of nine. Older children may need some standard hypnotherapy treatment in addition, to reinforce the improvement.

MIGRAINE

Migraine is an extremely common condition, affecting nearly one in five women and one in ten men. Over half of those who suffer from migraine have one or more attacks a month. Common symptoms include a pounding headache (which is usually one-sided and is made worse by movement), sensitivity to light and to noise, and nausea and vomiting. In some people, an attack is heralded by an 'aura'—a period of up to half an hour before the headache starts when the sufferer sees flashing lights or experiences dizziness, numbness or tingling and may find that her speech or hearing are affected in some way.

No one really knows what causes migraine but research has shown that it is caused by a change in the brain which results in it responding abnormally to normal sensory signals such as sensation, light or sound. For most people, drug treatment seems to be the only answer. But, for many, hypnotherapy can produce an equally satisfactory result.

If you suffer from migraine and decide to try hypnosis, the therapist will probably want to know the exact details of your attacks, so that specific suggestions can be given. But relaxation and general suggestions can also play a part.

You may be told, when you are in trance, that your attacks will become less frequent and less severe as you learn to relax more. This is likely to be helpful because tension can be a precipitating factor for migraine, and practicing self-hypnosis can help you to become more relaxed.

However, the therapist may also teach you a method by which you can cut short an impending attack. One such technique is for you to go into hypnosis and rest your hand against the painful area of your head. You then imagine a warmth flowing from your hand into your head, and this warmth will soothe and relax you. Slowly the warmth grows and begins to replace the pain. Eventually, you will no longer be aware of any pain in your head — it will all have been replaced by a comforting feeling of warmth which will remain for a little while after you wake from the trance. This method can work surprisingly quickly and even migraines that have been going on for several hours may respond.

Another useful technique is the 'clenched fist' which has already been discussed in the sections on anxiety and asthma. This is best used at the start of a migraine attack, so you may be taught both this and the 'warmth' method to cover all eventualities. It used to be thought that migraine was caused by the blood vessels of the brain contracting and dilating and, while this theory has now been superseded, the image is still a useful one to use. So you would be asked to shut your eyes and picture your brain, with all the blood vessels that run round it looking very constricted and constricting. First you would clench your fists to mirror this constriction, and then relax your hands, allowing the vessels to return to normal. It can equally well be done by picturing the tension in the muscles of the scalp and face and then helping them to relax by unclenching your fists. While the instructions for this will, of course, be given to you while you are in trance, you won't have to hypnotize yourself before using this technique so it is suitable to use under any circumstances.

SKIN CONDITIONS

It might be thought that, while hypnosis is appropriate to the treatment of conditions such as migraine, in which the symptoms are entirely functional, it would be far less likely to help those which appear to be purely physical in nature, such as eczema and psoriasis. But, in fact, both these conditions can respond extremely well, as can other skin conditions, as we shall see.

Psoriasis
Psoriasis is a condition in which skin cells build up to form raised 'plaques' that can be both itchy and unsightly. The plaques can form anywhere on the body but are frequently found on pressure areas such as the elbows and knees, as well as the back and scalp, where the constant shedding of scales can make it appear that the patient has severe dandruff.

For many years, the cause of psoriasis was a mystery but, in recent years, it has been discovered that it is what is known as an 'auto-immune' condition. In other words, a certain type of cell in the immune system becomes overactive and attacks healthy cells in the body. Other auto-immune conditions include celiac disease, multiple sclerosis, rheumatoid arthritis and ulcerative colitis.

Very often patients who suffer from psoriasis will notice that if they become upset or stressed, their skin will get worse. So treatment consists mainly of relaxation therapy, coupled with suggestions that the patches of psoriasis will become smaller and smaller until they disappear completely. Patients may also be given a visualization, to use when they are doing self-hypnosis, in which they can see their skin gradually becoming clearer and feel it becoming more comfortable.

Eczema
Eczema is a condition in which the skin becomes dry, scaly and itchy and, in severe cases, can split or become infected. Most cases can be classified as either 'atopic' or 'contact'. Contact eczema means that the condition has been caused by contact with an outside agent (such as nickel or strong disinfectant) and can normally be quickly cleared by removing the cause. Atopic eczema, however, is a long-term condition which usually begins in childhood. Sometimes patients will also suffer from asthma, and the condition may run in families.

The itch of eczema may be very hard for children to tolerate, and they may scratch themselves until they bleed. The constant discomfort may make children very fretful and irritable—a state of mind that is not going to facilitate healing so, here again, relaxation is the key.

When children are treated with hypnosis, no matter what the reason, it is vital that they feel secure. So suggestions are often given to them while they are in the trance that will help them feel safe and reassured that they will get better. A 'negative hallucination' may be induced by suggestions that the itching will become less intense and fade away. (A positive hallucination is one in which the patient feels, sees or hears something that isn't there; a negative hallucination is one in which he no longer feels, sees or hears something that is. A moderate to deep level of trance is necessary to induce either sort of hallucination but, fortunately, most children are good subjects.)

Whatever the condition that is being treated, the therapist needs to explain what is going to happen in terms that the patient can relate to. For example, in the case of eczema, the irritation may have been going on for so long that it may be impossible for a child to remember what it feels like for his skin not to be itchy. So the therapist will need to find out whether there is anything that relieves the condition, even partially. Perhaps the child has been using a steroid cream with some relief. In such a case, when he is being taught a technique, he might be told that it will relieve the itching just as much as the steroid cream—and perhaps a little bit more. Once the therapy has started to take effect, suggestions can be given that his skin will feel a little better each day. Finally, when the irritation is only minimal, a suggestion that it will stop completely will be accepted by the child's subconscious mind.

Most children are imaginative and can visualize without trouble. So, in the treatment of eczema, they may be asked to

155

imagine that they are swimming in a pool of warm water in a beautiful garden and that, as they swim, the water is helping their skin to heal. They can be told to look down through the crystal clear water and see that the rash is slowly fading.

Another method is to ask children to imagine that their hands are growing bigger and warmer, so that they become as big as tennis racquets. Once they have done this, they are asked to stroke the affected areas of their skin with their large, warm hands and are told that the heat will make more blood flow through the skin. They are told that the blood will carry with it the nutrition that the skin needs to get better. Then the children are asked to imagine their hands returning to normal size and becoming cold. Again they stroke the affected areas and, this time, they are told that the coldness will seal in the healing properties of the blood so that the skin will continue to improve, even after they wake up from hypnosis. Once they have learned them, either of these visualization techniques can be used by children when they practice self-hypnosis.

Extraordinary results with a rare skin condition
In 1952, Dr. Albert A. Mason, an anesthetist and hypnotherapist, was working at the Queen Victoria Hospital in East Grinstead, Sussex—a hospital which had become famous for pioneering the use of plastic surgery for badly injured or burned airmen during World War II. Quite a few of the doctors who train as hypnotherapists are anesthetists, because hypnosis can be a valuable tool in pain clinics (which are often run by anasthetists). But Dr. Mason didn't use hypnosis just for the control of pain. He had been successful in treating other conditions, too, and had managed to help a number of patients to get rid of warts.

One day, Dr. Mason saw a young man of 16 who had come into hospital to have skin grafts. He was covered in what appeared to be the worst case of warts the anesthetist had ever seen—his skin was covered in a black horny substance and this had cracked and become chronically infected. Dr. Mason asked the surgeon whether hypnosis had been considered, since warts could respond well. The surgeon gave him a scathing look and suggested that, if he wanted to, he could try treating the patient.

Dr. Mason took the suggestion at face value and hypnotized the young man. He told him that the warts on his left arm were going to fall off. And, five days later, the horny layer on that arm softened and fell off, leaving normal-looking skin underneath. Dr. Mason called the surgeon in to see this, but was not prepared for his reaction. The surgeon was flabbergasted—because this was not a bad case of warts. The patient had a congenital condition—ichthyosiform erythrodermia of Brocq—which was incurable. He had already had two unsuccessful skin grafts—the grafted skin had just become as black and horny as the rest.

An explanation for this extraordinary result was sought. But it seemed impossible because patients with this condition don't just have a horny layer covering their body—they actually lack the oil-producing glands that keep normal skin soft and allow it to renew itself. Years later, in an interview, Dr. Mason theorized that there were tiny undeveloped remnants of these glands in the patient's skin and that the suggestions given under hypnosis must have somehow stimulated them to grow.

But what happened after this was equally inexplicable. Having achieved success with the patient's left arm, Dr. Mason treated his right arm, then his legs and, finally, his trunk. The results on his legs were not as good as on his arms, but still were enough to allow him to start living a normal life which, previously, had been impossible. Three years later, Dr. Mason caught up with the patient and found that none of the treated areas had relapsed. There were, however, still a few black patches here and there. But when Dr. Mason attempted to treat them, he found that the patient was now 'totally unhypnotizable'.

After this, he found another eight patients with the same condition and offered to treat them with hypnosis. But the therapy had no effect on any of them. However, round about the same time, a doctor in Oxford, who had read of Mason's success, treated two sisters, aged five and seven, who had the same condition and managed to improve their skin considerably.

Why some patients should have responded well to hypnosis and others not at all has not been explained. Guy Lyon Playfair, in his book *If This be Magic: the Forgotten Power of Hypnosis*, suggests that it is a reflection of the therapist's confidence and belief in his ability to make a difference. Dr. Mason thought that the first patient had warts—and he knew that he had successfully treated warts. But, after three years, it is possible that knowledge of the actual diagnosis—and the fact that the condition was 'incurable'—had influenced him subconsciously so that he was no longer as confident that he could clear up the remaining patches, or treat the other eight patients. The Oxford doctor, however, had read a report of Dr. Mason's first case, knew that it could be done—and did it.

NOCTURNAL ENURESIS (BED WETTING)

Up to the age of about five, children are still learning how to control their bladders and bed wetting is not considered to be abnormal. Assessments vary but probably between 15 and 30 per cent of five year olds still wet at night and five per cent of ten year olds. It tends to be more common in boys than in girls. Some form of treatment may be necessary once a child has reached school age, or even earlier if wetting occurs more often than once or twice a week.

Bed wetting can cause great stress in a family. Because tension can make the condition worse, parents are always advised to refrain from punishing the child and to reassure him that it is not his fault. But a parent who has to wash sheets five, six or seven times a week is apt to become a little short-tempered. Eventually she may start to feel that the child really could control himself if he wanted to and that either he is continuing to wet because he is too lazy to get up to go to the toilet or because, for some reason, he wants to punish her.

If there are other children in the family, they may get upset by the situation, too. They may resent the fact that their mother is always irritable. If they share a room with the child who wets, they may object to the fact that the room often smells of urine. And if the wetting makes it impossible for the family to go on holiday, this is bound to cause tensions.

In a case such as this, it may be necessary to treat both the parent and the child. The parent can be taught to relax in order to cope better with the problem, and the child, who is frustrated and miserable due to his inability to stop wetting, can be given a technique whereby he can help himself.

There are, of course, orthodox methods of treatment available. The 'alarm' method is popular and effective for a lot of children. The mechanism is attached to the bed and, if it becomes damp, it rings a bell or a buzzer, waking the child at the very moment that he starts to urinate. Eventually, he becomes so used to waking when he wants to pass water, that he can do so automatically without the aid of the alarm.

However, some children do not react to the alarms but manage to sleep through them. For these, some medication may be recommended. Of the drugs available, imipramine has probably been around the longest. But, because of possible side effects and the fact that it tends only to work for as long as the child is taking it, it is not the treatment of first choice. Desmopressin is more commonly prescribed and it acts by reducing the amount of urine the kidneys produce, so that the child's bladder becomes less full.

Up to the age of about six, there is still a good chance that the child will stop bed wetting of his own accord, so children under this age are not usually treated by any method. Children aged six or seven may be treated with hypnotherapy if they are well motivated—which, on the whole, they are. They dislike the fact that they wet their beds just as much as their parents do, and are just as anxious to find something that will stop it.

The keynote to the treatment of a child with enuresis is reassurance. While in hypnosis, he must be reassured that his parents love him, even though they may sometimes get cross with him. He must be reassured that the bedwetting is not his fault and that there is no reason for him to feel guilty about it. And he must be reassured that it will stop in due course.

He may be told that there are many things that his body does for itself without him having to think about them — things such as breathing and digesting food. But, whereas the lungs automatically know how to breathe and the stomach knows how to digest, the bladder has to learn how to control passing water. In his case, it has obviously learned how to do it most of the time, because when he is awake he doesn't wet himself and he can go a long time without having to pass water. Now the treatment that he is going to be given will teach the bladder how to behave at night. And once it has learned, it will never forget.

The child is told that the reason he wets at night is because the bladder lets go of the water it's holding long before it's full. He is asked to think of his bladder as being like a balloon, which is able to stretch so that it can hold lots of water — as it does during the day. He is asked to put a hand on his abdomen and to picture his bladder stretching. As he does so, he is told that he will start to feel that he wants to pass water. When the sensation starts, he is to say to his bladder "You're not full" and this will remind his bladder that, during the day, it can hold much more, so the feeling will go away.

The child is told that if he practices this technique when he is doing his self-hypnosis, his bladder will remember how much water it can hold. And, because he is constantly reminding it, it will remember, even when he is asleep, that there is no need to pass water until it is full. As a precaution, he will be told that if his bladder does become full during the night, he will wake up and go to the toilet, rather than wetting the bed. Finally, he is told that his bladder is very clever and will probably start to learn what to do quite quickly, so within a short time he should be having many more dry nights.

For many children, a technique such as this will be all they need. But some have deep-rooted reasons for continuing to wet and, for these, some form of hypnoanalysis or psychotherapy may be necessary. This is not possible for very young children but older children may reveal problems that have been suppressed and that are manifesting as enuresis.

If the patient is in his teens, enuresis is harder to treat. If the condition has continued to this age, there is usually some underlying reason, and this may be hard to elicit. Adolescents may be poor hypnotic subjects and so investigation of their anxieties and emotions may need psychotherapy rather than hypnotherapy. It is also possible that there may be some secondary gain from the enuresis (that is, the patient may actually be benefiting in some way from continuing to wet the bed) and subconsciously he may not wish to stop. If it is possible to discover the root cause, the patient can be helped to understand and acknowledge it, so that he can learn to express his emotions in another way.

PAIN

The induction of a 'negative hallucination' (mentioned in the section on eczema) can be very valuable for the treatment of chronic pain. However, the use of hypnosis to control pain is fraught with danger and should never be used by anyone who is not a doctor or dentist. It is certainly not something that patients with an ability to do self-hypnosis should try for themselves. The danger is, of course, obvious when you think about it. If you routinely use hypnosis to remove pain, then it's all too easy to mask a potentially life-threatening condition, such as an inflamed appendix.

The therapist must therefore be absolutely sure that the patient's pain has been fully investigated and has been shown to be safe to treat, and he must also ensure that the patient, once taught to use the technique, will be unable to use it for any other type of pain.

Before teaching an adult this technique, the therapist will explain the dangers of masking undiagnosed pain. Children may be unable to understand this, or may not remember it so, as a general rule, they are not taught how to use self-hypnosis to alleviate pain. However, it is perfectly possible for a dentist, for example, to use hypnosis on a child during treatment and so lessen the need for local anaesthetic, without actually having to teach the child how to use pain control.

Adults who are taught how to control pain will be given a post-hypnotic suggestion that they will only be able to use the technique under very specific circumstances. Other safeguards will also be included. For example, a patient who suffers from migraine or from tension headaches may be taught how to control this pain. But it is possible that she may then develop a severe headache that is due to another cause (such as high blood pressure) and may misinterpret this symptom as being the headache from which she usually suffers. Masking this headache may lead to diagnosis, and therefore treatment, being delayed. So she will be given the suggestion that the pain control that she can induce will only be effective for the length of time her migraines usually last. If the pain is still there when the effect wears off, it may be an indication to consult a doctor.

A similar suggestion will also be used for patients who are taught self-hypnosis by their dentists. The removal of pain may be an extremely useful technique if you suddenly develop toothache at eleven o'clock on a Sunday night, but if you continue to control the pain rather than go to the dentist, you may end up with a seriously infected mouth.

One simple method of pain relief has already been mentioned in the section on migraine—that of replacing the pain with a feeling of warmth. A useful method for dental treatment approaches pain control from the opposite direction, based on the idea that loss of feeling can be caused by cold.

Having been hypnotized, the patient is asked to imagine that, next to his chair, there is a bucket containing some water and a lot of ice. When he can picture it clearly, he is asked to put his hand into the bucket. The therapist continues to talk

164

to the patient, telling him how cold his hand is becoming and how he is losing the feeling in it. Finally, the patient is told to take his hand out of the bucket and to pinch it with his other hand. In this way, he proves to himself that his hand is really numb, because he can't feel the pinch. Then he is told to lift his hand and place it against that part of his mouth in which the dental treatment is to take place. Gradually, he will be aware that the numbness is transferring from his hand to his mouth, and his hand is regaining sensation while his mouth becomes completely numb. Finally he is told that, when the treatment is carried out, he will not feel it, any more than he was able to feel himself pinching his hand.

Another method, requiring a more detailed visualization, is one in which the patient is asked to imagine an old-fashioned telephone switchboard. He is told that this switchboard represents his brain. Wires are plugged in all over it, linking his brain to different parts of his body. And next to each wire socket is an on/off switch with a little light. If the switch is at 'on', the light will be on. If the switch is turned off, the light will go off. Each switch has a label under it saying which part of the body it is connected to, and the patient is asked to look for the socket and switch that are connected to the painful area which is to be treated. For example, if the patient has an ingrowing toenail on his right big toe, he looks for a label saying 'right big toe'.

Once he has found it, he is asked to make sure that it is the correct socket by checking that the switch and the light are both on. To make the visualization more vivid, he is asked to say what color the light is and what color the wire is that is plugged into the socket. He is then asked to turn the switch off and unplug the wire, and he is told that, in doing so, he has cut off the nervous link between his brain and his right big toe. So it is now impossible for any pain signals to get through to his brain and, as a result, the pain in his toe will disappear.

The anesthesia that the patient feels as a result of this technique will be very localized and it is therefore a useful alternative to local anesthetic in suitable patients. Another method is to suggest to the patient that he is having a local anesthetic injected into the painful area. You may wonder why this method should be any better than actually giving a local anesthetic but, as you will know if you've ever had one, the anesthetizing injection itself can be quite painful. When, in hypnosis, you visualize having such an injection, you don't imagine the pain associated with it, but only the resulting numbness.

In order to be able to produce any form of hallucination, a patient needs to be able to go into a medium depth or deep trance, so those people who are 'light' subjects may be unable to develop a sufficient degree of anesthesia on its own for minor operations or dental treatment to be performed. However, the technique can still be useful. Even a moderate degree of numbness can prevent the injection of a local anesthetic from being unpleasant, and may reduce the amount of anesthetic that is needed.

Even patients who cannot develop any useful degree of anesthesia may benefit from being told that "any pain you feel will not worry or upset you". This can be a very important suggestion, since the emotional content of pain can add greatly to its unpleasantness. It is well known that some types of pain are much more unpleasant than others, even though they may be of equal intensity. It is perfectly possible for patients to endure quite severe pain if the emotional aspect has been removed.

A further benefit of hypnosis in pain control is, once again, its ability to help the patient relax. Very often, chronic pain can become a vicious cycle, with the pain making the patient tense and the tension intensifying the pain. If the patient can be taught to relax rather than tense up when he feels the pain coming on, the pain may be reduced dramatically.

Terminally ill patients can be treated quite safely with hypnosis and so avoid the side-effects of heavy medication with analgesic drugs, the doses of which can thus be reduced. Patients who have intermittent pain, if they are capable of inducing a hallucination, may be taught the technique of time distortion, so that it appears to them that time passes very quickly when they are in pain, and slows down again to normal between attacks.

TINNITUS

Tinnitus, or ringing in the ears, is a most unpleasant condition, usually occurring in older people and often associated with deafness. The patient is aware of a constant buzzing, hum, or other sound, sometimes predominantly in one ear, which may be so distressing that it dominates his life. Orthodox medicine has little to offer in the treatment of tinnitus but, fortunately, other therapies such as acupuncture, homeopathy and hypnotherapy, may be able to relieve the patient's symptoms.

The hypnotherapeutic treatment involves the production of a negative hallucination, and so is less likely to be of use for those patients who are only capable of going into a very light trance. However, because a constant noise in the ears and an inability to hear clearly may be very demoralizing, ego-strengthening techniques may benefit any patient with tinnitus and this, of course, can be done at any depth of trance.

In the same way that a patient can be taught to remove pain, so someone with tinnitus can be taught to remove the ringing. Since there is no danger involved in masking the noise, no time limit need be put on the effect and the patient can be taught to use the technique himself, so as to maintain the hallucination if it should start to wear off.

A useful method is to ask the patient to visualize an old-fashioned radio, with large knobs and dials. When he can see it clearly, he is told that it is this that controls his tinnitus.

If he looks closely, he can see that the 'volume' knob is turned up high and the needle on the dial next to it is showing almost maximum volume. It is often more effective to start with a positive hallucination of an increase in the noise before starting to decrease it. So the patient is asked to move the volume knob slightly, so that the noise in his ears increases a fraction and the dial moves up even further. When he has done this, he is asked to turn the knob back to where it was before, and hear the noise decrease.

Once the tinnitus is back to its normal level, the patient is asked to start to turn the knob down very gently. It is important that this is done gradually in order to allow the patient to feel that he has complete control over what he is doing. At the first session, therefore, the tinnitus may be reduced slightly, but it may be some time before it has completely disappeared. However, if the patient is willing to practice self-hypnosis regularly, this may speed up the process so that it is not too long before the tinnitus is considerably reduced from its original level. As the noise decreases, the patient will gain confidence in his own ability to control it and this, in itself, will make the later stages of treatment easier.

It may be necessary for the patient to continue to do regular daily self-hypnosis for the rest of his life in order to keep his tinnitus under control, but most patients would consider this a small price to pay to get rid of this unpleasant condition.

169

PHOBIAS

A phobia is an irrational fear of a particular thing. Quite often, the sufferer knows that the fear is foolish but, despite this, can do nothing about it. Mild phobias such as fear of spiders or of mice are fairly common but it is usually possible to live with them without too much difficulty. However, a severe phobia can disrupt the patient's life, because he will spend all his time worrying about and trying to avoid the object of his fear.

The commonest phobia for which treatment is requested is agoraphobia (fear of open spaces) which is commoner in women than in men and may prevent the patient from even being able to set foot outside her home. Then comes fear of illness or of death, followed by fear of other people or of animals. Other fairly common phobias are acrophobia (fear of heights), nyctophobia (fear of the dark) and claustrophobia (fear of small spaces). Less common ones include fear of water, fear of fire, fear of thunderstorms, fear of insanity, fear of snakes, and fear of cats. And fear of doctors and dentists is not uncommon!

Hypnotherapy can be used in a variety of ways. Firstly, patients must be given adequate ego-strengthening techniques, because the feeling that your life is being ruled by a ridiculous and unnecessary fear can be very demoralizing. They need to be able to develop confidence in themselves and in their ability to conquer whatever phobias are troubling them.

Sometimes all that is needed to overcome a phobia is a simple visualization technique. For example, if the patient is a woman suffering from agoraphobia who is unable to go outside her house without feeling panic, she might be asked to visualize herself inside her front door and about to open it. Very slowly, she opens the door and stands looking out, but not stepping over the threshold. The hypnotherapist reassures her that she is quite safe—she is still in her house and she can shut the door at any time she wants to. She may be given a technique by which she can rid herself of any tension or anxiety which is beginning to build up. This may be something similar to the 'clenched fist' technique described in the section on anxiety, in which the patient can throw away her tension with her hands and breathe it out through her lungs. Or it may be a phrase which she can repeat to herself, such as 'calm and relaxed' or 'safe and secure'.

Once the patient can picture herself standing at the open door without feeling any tension, she is asked to step out of the house. Again she stops and controls any tension or anxiety before going further. Next, she may take two or three steps, stopping only if she feels anxious. Because the visualization has to be taken very slowly, it may take quite a long time before the patient can even get to her own garden gate, but her confidence will be increasing all the time.

Self-hypnosis is very important and the patient will need to practice regularly. In order to give her added confidence when she is using the visualization technique on her own, she may be told that, if she feels anxious, the visualization will 'freeze', just as if she has stopped a film from running. Not only will she stay still, but she will find that her anxiety

171

is cut short. She can then use whatever technique she likes to ensure that she is relaxed and, when she is ready, can start the film running again, either from where she was or else, if she prefers, from the beginning.

The more often the patient visualizes herself performing, and coping with, the action which previously brought on uncontrollable panic, the more confident she will become that she can do it in real life. She will start to have faith in her relaxation techniques which, the therapist will have assured her, will be just as effective when she confronts her phobia for real as they are when she is in hypnosis. It is often a slow process, but patients who were previously unable to get out of the house may eventually be able to enjoy a normal life again.

In some cases, the patient may not respond, possibly because the phobia resulted from some very traumatic incident whose memory is still being stored, but suppressed, by the subconscious mind. In cases like this, some hypnoanalysis or psychotherapy will be needed to try to discover the original cause of the phobia. The techniques used in hypnoanalysis are similar to those mentioned in the chapter on regression and, indeed, regression may be very helpful in the treatment of phobias.

THE USE OF HYPNOSIS IN CHILDBIRTH

There is no doubt that a woman who has attended ante-natal relaxation classes is far more likely to have an easy labor than one who has not. Ideally, the mother should be able to relax between contractions and, during the second stage of labor, should be able to use her contractions so that she pushes with them and does not struggle against them. It follows, therefore, that the relaxation induced by hypnosis should be of benefit to a mother in labor. However, hypnosis has far more to offer a pregnant woman than mere relaxation.

Over the years, pediatricians have become increasingly concerned about the effect of pain-killing drugs, given during labor, on the newborn baby. Mothers, too, are aware of this problem and many now opt for 'natural childbirth'. Unfortunately, even when a woman is fully prepared for her labor, she may still need to be given pain-killers. But a patient using hypnosis may be able to control her pain to such an extent that she can either make do with a very small dose or do without drugs altogether. She will, of course, need to start her hypnotherapy sessions quite early on in her pregnancy so that, by the time she goes into labor, she has had adequate practice in the various techniques that she will need to use.

She will not be taught to anesthetize her pain completely but, rather, will be told that any pain she feels during labor will be tolerable and will not worry her. This is very important. One of the complaints which may be expressed by women who have given birth with the help of an epidural (an injection into the spinal column which anesthetizes all the body below the level of that injection) is that they did not feel that they were taking part in the delivery of their children. If pain is completely absent, then the work seems to have been done entirely by the obstetrician or midwife, and the mother is left feeling vaguely unsatisfied and as though she has somehow missed out on this important experience.

It is, of course, important that someone should be present at the delivery who can help the mother with her hypnosis. Some therapists invite the midwife or obstetric nurse to attend the ante-natal hypnotherapy sessions so that she can give the appropriate instructions and suggestions when the patient is in labor. Some obstetricians practise hypnosis and offer it to their patients. The main problem with using hypnosis is that it is time-consuming for the hypnotherapist who has to run the ante-natal sessions. However, it would seem that this is time well spent when mothers come through their deliveries with ease and when the risk of their babies being affected by sedatives and pain-killers is removed.

THE USE OF HYPNOSIS IN DENTISTRY

Hypnosis can be used in a variety of ways in a dental practice. It can calm down those patients who are afraid to have treatment. It can be used to dull pain, instead of, or together with, local anesthesia. And, for work that is going to take some time, suggestions can be given to the patient that the time will seem to pass very quickly.

For people who have a dental phobia, the dentist will need to see them, for the first few sessions at least, outside the room in which the treatment will be given. Some dentists who use hypnosis will have a separate room for this. Otherwise it may be necessary for the patient to see another hypnotherapist and then be passed on to the dentist once the fear of entering his office has been reduced.

The treatment of this problem is along the same lines as that of other phobias. And, of course, the dentist doesn't have to be a hypnotherapist. Like Dr. James Bramwell (see chapter two) the therapist only has to tell the dentist the key phrases necessary for him to be able to put a 'primed' patient into hypnosis and, once in a trance, the patient can do the rest.

For a patient who wishes to avoid having injections for dental treatment, the numbing effect of the 'hand in the bucket of ice' technique can be used, as described in the section on pain. Since this technique may take quite a time before complete analgesia occurs, the hypnotherapist would need to teach the patient how to use self-hypnosis so that he can practice at home for a few weeks before coming for treatment.

CHAPTER EIGHT: SOME AUTHENTIC CASE HISTORIES

The cases described in this chapter are all those of patients whom I have treated personally. Their names and personal details have been changed to ensure their privacy.

SAM

Sam was a policeman who had failed his promotion examinations on two occasions. If he failed a third time, the likelihood was that he wouldn't be allowed to take them again. As the examination dates drew nearer, he was becoming very anxious particularly with regard to one particular subject that he had always had difficulties with. Now his anxiety was interfering with his ability to recall information and, no matter how much he read about this subject, it just wasn't sinking in.

First of all, I taught Sam how to use self-hypnosis in order to relax. I suggested that he use it every day for 15 minutes just before he started his revision. While he was in hypnosis, I also told him that if he repeated the formula 'calm and relaxed' a few times every 15 minutes or so while he was studying, he would stop himself from tensing up. But if he did start to feel tension, he could relieve it by taking a deep breath and breathing the tension out. I gave him several ego-strengthening suggestions, finishing by telling him that there was no reason why he should not pass these exams, because it was only his anxiety that was holding him back, not his ability.

Once he had practiced these techniques and was beginning to take a more relaxed attitude towards his studies, I gave Sam the suggestion that, if he recorded all the information that he wanted to learn and played it back to himself while he was practicing his self-hypnosis, he would retain a great deal of it. He started to use this method and, a few weeks later, was able to pass his exams without difficulty.

CLAUDIA

Claudia was a 42 year old mother of two who had been suffering from psoriasis for about seven years. At first, only her elbows and knees had been affected but, in the past two years, larger areas had become involved. She was very aware of the unsightly patches on her elbows and legs and so had taken to wearing long sleeves and thick stockings, even when the weather was hot. She also had some involvement of her scalp, so that it looked as though she had heavy dandruff and, as result, she had given up wearing dark clothes. Her mother had quite a severe form of psoriasis and Claudia was worried that her condition, too, would become widespread.

Although she wasn't a naturally anxious person, Claudia did have some stresses in her life. She admitted that there was sometimes tension between her husband and herself. He was an executive in a large company and often came home late from work, tired and bad-tempered. She had a fairly demanding part-time job and, what with that and looking after her home and her children, she was often tired by the time her husband arrived home. She sometimes had to 'bite her tongue' in order to avoid arguing with him, but then

177

would seethe inwardly because she hadn't told him what was on her mind. She was very much aware that the resulting tension—or any other emotional stress—would make her psoriasis worse.

At her first session, I gave Claudia ego-strengthening suggestions and taught her how to hypnotize herself. I told her that she would become very relaxed in everyday life and able to cope easily with everything that she had to do, and that minor traumas wouldn't upset her. I told her that, gradually, even her skin would relax and this would allow it to obtain more nourishment from the blood and to heal itself. I asked her to do regular self-hypnosis, in which she visualized the patches of psoriasis getting smaller and smaller until, eventually, they disappeared.

When she came for her second session, Claudia told me that she had been practicing self-hypnosis every day and was feeling more relaxed. However, she didn't feel that she was going very deeply into hypnosis when at home. I reassured her that this was not important.

She continued to improve, becoming far less tense and she began to realize that some of the tension at home had come from her. Now that she was more relaxed, her husband seemed to her to be less bad-tempered!

Claudia had five sessions of hypnotherapy, at intervals of about ten days, after which her psoriasis had completely disappeared. I advised her to continue with her self-hypnosis every day, visualizing her skin remaining clear and unblemished, and to return if she had any problems.

She returned just once, eight months later, when a very small patch of psoriasis had appeared after an emotional upset. This disappeared after one session and I didn't see her again.

JOSHUA

When he left school, Joshua joined the Army. He loved the active life and, being intelligent and capable, it didn't take him long to rise to the rank of sergeant. However, his Army career was cut short when he was posted to Afghanistan and, only weeks after his arrival, was badly injured. He was in hospital for several months and, eventually, had to have his right leg amputated.

Being young and resilient, he soon learned to walk again, using a prosthesis (false leg) but missed being able to play football. After he was discharged from the Army, he found a job with a company in the City of London, where his intelligence and capacity for hard work meant that, once again, he was able to move up the career ladder.

After his leg was amputated, Joshua had had intermittent pain in the stump but, at first, it wasn't too bad. However, over the years, it got worse, coming on if he had walked a great deal, and sometimes appearing when he was relaxing in the evening after a busy day.

He lived in Sussex, near the coast, and had to commute every day. Sometimes he wasn't able to get a seat on the train into London, nor on the underground train which took him to the City. He then had a six-minute walk from the station

179

to his office—and he often arrived in great pain. And the same thing might happen on the way home in the evening, although he was inclined to leave work late in order to miss the worst of the rush-hour. But this, of course, meant that he was having less time to spend with his family.

Joshua had consulted his doctor frequently about the problem. He had been back to the Limb Centre on numerous occasions and various types of prosthesis had been tried, but none seemed better than any other. His doctor had also referred him to a surgeon and to a neurologist, but no one had been able to help him. Although he had pain-killers that he could take when he needed them, he tried to avoid using them when he was at work because he found they made him a bit sleepy and impaired his concentration—although not taking them was just as bad because when the pain was very severe it stopped him from focusing on his work.

He described the pain as being cramp-like and he was aware that it occurred more often when he was particularly busy or under pressure at work. It could come on quite suddenly and, sometimes, would last for two or three days without any let-up. In the six months before he came to see me, he had been experiencing pain every day, and it was gradually getting worse and worse. Not only that, but when he took pain-killers they no longer seemed as effective as they had been in the past.

There are different types of pain that can be experienced by amputees. One of these is 'phantom limb pain' which usually occurs immediately after the amputation and seems to the patient to be coming from the limb that is no longer there, often from the farthest part—the foot or the hand. This type of pain can be treated with hypnotherapy and trials have shown that around 80 per cent of patients experience considerable or complete relief. However, Joshua didn't have phantom limb pain—he was feeling pain in the stump itself. There was no soreness or redness on the skin surface, so clearly the pain wasn't being caused by an ill-fitting prosthesis. The only alternative seemed to be that it was due to some form of muscle spasm.

With this diagnosis in mind, Joshua's doctor suggested he try some hypnosis. Joshua agreed, although he was doubtful as to whether it could help. However, on the grounds that it couldn't do any harm, he made an appointment to see me.

Fortunately, he was a good hypnotic subject and went easily into the depth of trance needed to induce pain relief. At the first session, I taught him self-hypnosis and asked him to practice it every day for two weeks, before coming back for his second appointment. I also taught him a variation of the 'clenched fist' technique (described in the section on anxiety in chapter seven) to try to relieve some of the spasm that seemed to be occurring in the muscles of his stump.

At his second session, Joshua told me that he had been determined to let the therapy work if it possibly could and had practiced his self-hypnosis quite successfully for about three days. But then, for no apparent reason, he had "lost the knack" and, although he continued to practice, he had been unable to put himself into trance. It seemed as though the reason for this was that he didn't yet have adequate confidence in his ability to use the techniques that he had learned, so we went through these again.

In addition, I introduced the 'telephone switchboard' visualization technique (described in the section on pain relief in chapter seven). Joshua found it hard to visualize the switchboard but agreed to practice it for a week to see whether it became any easier (as often happens). Unfortunately, although it did become somewhat easier over the week for him to picture the switchboard and to 'turn off' the appropriate link to his leg, this only eased the pain slightly.

So, in the next session, I taught him the 'bucket of ice' technique (described in the section on pain relief) and he found this much easier. As soon as his hand went numb, I asked him to place it on his stump, over the painful area. I gave him suggestions that the numbness would flow from his hand into the stump, deadening the pain, while the feeling in his hand would return to normal. The smile that spread across his face showed me that the suggestion was taking effect!

While he was still in hypnosis, I told Joshua that this pain relief would be long-lasting. If he felt that it was wearing off, he could 'top it up' by repeating the technique. I suggested that he routinely went through the technique two or three times a week, while doing his self-hypnosis, in order to maintain the analgesic effect at a constant level. It was safe to do this because this was a long-term condition of which the cause was known. However, there was always a possibility that other pain caused, for example, by his skin being rubbed by his prosthesis, or by an infection, could occur in this area. So I continued by saying "This is a very special kind of numbness. It will deaden only the pain from which you have been suffering for so many years, and on that it will be very effective. But it will have no effect whatsoever on any other pain that occurs in the stump. Nor will it have any effect on any pain occurring anywhere else in your body." When Joshua woke up from the trance, he said that the pain had gone.

After this session he was able to control the pain quite successfully. He found that it was reduced by the initial relaxation and then what remained was fairly easily removed using the 'ice bucket' technique. However, once again, he seemed to lose confidence in himself after about five days and, while he could still put himself in hypnosis, he couldn't get the pain control to work. When he came for his next appointment, I reinforced the techniques that I had taught him previously and I gave him suggestions that he would start to feel very confident in his ability to use them.

Three weeks later, Joshua returned in a very jubilant state. He had had hardly any pain since his last session and he had been able to control the small amount that had occurred by using the 'ice bucket' technique. His only complaint was that he hadn't discovered hypnotherapy sooner.

Joshua had only one more session of treatment. This was about two years later, when he requested an appointment to reinforce what he had previously been taught. He had had a very busy few months and had allowed his self-hypnosis practice to lapse. The pain had just started to come back and he was a little concerned in case he had lost the knack of dealing with it. However, when I saw him, it was clear to me that he was still perfectly capable of controlling the pain and just needed reassurance and a reminder to practice his self-hypnosis as often as he could.

DONNA

Donna was a 26 year old woman who came to see me "as a last resort" to try to get some relief from back pain. It had started about six years previously when she had strained herself doing some heavy lifting. The pain had died down but then recurred at frequent intervals and, in the three years before she saw me, the episodes had become longer and the pain-free periods between them had become shorter.

Donna had been married for three years and she and her husband would have liked to have started a family, but she felt she could not go through a pregnancy in her present state of health. When she was in pain, she found she was unable to do housework, cooking or shopping. Sometimes she was incapacitated for a week or more and she became very distressed when she had to rely on her husband to do the things which she considered to be her responsibility. Recently, she had started to believe that, eventually, the pain would be constant and she would be confined to a wheelchair, which would make her quite unable to look after a family. She felt depressed and demoralized. She longed to be more active but, even between attacks, had to be extremely careful not to over-exert herself in case the exercise triggered off another attack.

When she first hurt her back, Donna's doctor referred her for some physiotherapy. She had found this helpful to begin with but, after the pain had recurred for the third or fourth time, the treatment no longer seemed to have any effect. Some three or four years later she tried osteopathy but did not find it helpful.

When she first came to see me, she was taking a lot of pain-killers on a regular basis. She told me that, as soon as the pain started, she "knew" that she was going to have several days of severe pain. She had always tended to be a worrier and, for the past year or two, had been suffering from tension headaches which, like the back pain, had been getting increasingly frequent and now occurred about once a week.

As I listened to her tell her story, it became clear to me that what was uppermost in her mind was the fear of being confined to a wheelchair and in constant pain for the rest of her life. I began to wonder whether it might be possible to do a little more for her than just give her a technique to relieve the pain because, if tension was a major factor, teaching her to relax should help. However, since she had had so little relief from other therapies, I doubted whether hypnosis could relieve her symptoms entirely.

Fortunately, Donna was a good subject and went into hypnosis readily. After the initial deepening and ego-strengthening techniques, I gave her suggestions that she had nothing to fear — that her back would not get worse and that she would not finish up in a wheelchair. I told her that she was in the process of learning to relax and that knowing how to do this would make her life easier. Even when she was not completely free of pain, the fact that she could relax would make it easier for her to cope and to carry on with her life.

Then I taught her self-hypnosis and a progressive relaxation technique. This technique is sometimes used to deepen the patient's trance at the start of a session and is one which a lot of people use, without hypnosis, to help them get to sleep. There are several versions, but in this case I asked her to imagine that a flood of golden light was pouring down onto the top of her head and was flowing down through her body and around it, bathing her with warmth and relaxation. As she did so, I asked her to concentrate on each group of muscles in turn and to feel them relax, starting with the muscles of the scalp, then the forehead, the face and the jaw. (Good subjects may drop the jaw to such an extent that the movement can be seen by the therapist sitting several feet away.)

Then I asked Donna to concentrate on the muscles of her neck, feeling them relax as they were bathed in the golden light. After this, I turned her attention to her shoulders (usually tense, even in the most relaxed person) and to her arms and I asked her to imagine that she was becoming loose and floppy like a rag doll. I asked her to relax all the large muscles of her chest — and, as with the relaxation of the jaw, the effect of this can sometimes be visible to the therapist. In normal breathing, the chest cavity is made larger and smaller by the movement of the muscles of the chest wall and of the diaphragm, the large sheet of muscle that divides the chest from the abdomen. When we are completely relaxed, we tend to breathe more with the diaphragm and it may be possible to see this change to diaphragmatic breathing when the patient consciously relaxes the chest muscles.

Because she was already very anxious about her back, there was the possibility that mentioning it, with a suggestion to relax it, might make Donna more tense rather than less. So, without using the word 'relax', I just asked her to feel the warm golden light flooding over her back, soothing it and making it more comfortable. I suggested that she would feel herself sinking into the chair (the use of the word 'sinking' also suggests that the patient will go deeper into trance). Finally, I asked her to relax the muscles of her abdomen, her legs and her feet.

Once she had gone through this progressive relaxation, I suggested to Donna that she just sit and enjoy being in hypnosis. After a few minutes I asked her whether she felt any different from before. She said that the pain, which had been quite bad when she arrived for her appointment, was slightly less. This gave me something on which I could base my next set of suggestions.

I told her that the reason for the pain easing slightly was that she was more relaxed than she had been previously. I reminded her that, earlier, I had told her that learning to relax would help to relieve the pain and, already, she was seeing that this was true. In fact, I had not told her this. What I had said was that learning to relax would help her to cope with the pain, which is somewhat different. However, as it now seemed that relaxation was having an effect on the pain level, I could change the suggestion. Fortunately, it is possible to do this in hypnosis without troubling the patient, who will usually accept the most recent statement as being accurate.

I went on to tell Donna that a part of her pain was due to spasm in her back muscles. It might be a large part or a small part—only time would tell. But, since spasm can be relieved by relaxation and since, with practice, she would learn to relax enough to get rid of all the spasm, there was no doubt that she would be able to relieve at least part of her pain. I told her that the spasm was part of a vicious cycle—when the pain started she became tense and anxious because she was worried that she would not be able to look after her home and her family, and she was scared that, this time, the pain would be here to stay and she would finish up in a wheelchair. The tension and the anxiety naturally made themselves felt in the place where she was most susceptible—in her back. And so, the more worried she got, the more spasm there was in her back muscles—and this worried her even more. Now that she knew that some of the pain was due to spasm and that, by relaxing, she could relieve the spasm and reduce the pain, there was no longer any need for her to become tense or anxious when the pain came on. I also told her that the relaxation would help to control her headaches which, as she already knew, were due to tension.

188

Finally, I taught her a variation of the 'clenched fist' technique (described in the section on anxiety in chapter seven). I suggested that, as soon as the pain came on—either in her back or her head—she should lie down, shut her eyes, clench her fists tightly and then very slowly relax them, visualizing, at the same time, the relaxation of the back or head muscles that had gone into spasm. She should then follow this up by visualizing the golden light and using the progressive relaxation technique. I recommended that she practice self-hypnosis at least once a day—and more frequently if she had time—and that, on each occasion, she should go through the progressive relaxation technique.

I saw Donna again two weeks later. I asked her first about her headaches since it seemed likely that the lesser ailment might have started to respond to treatment, even if there hadn't yet been any improvement in her back pain. She said that she had had two headaches, one of which she had been able to control. I said that this was an encouraging start and asked whether she had noticed any improvement at all in her back. "Oh yes," she said. "It's much better." She had had only one attack of pain since her last session. When it started, she was aware that she didn't experience her usual feelings of anxiety and distress and she was able to control it with the techniques that she had learned. She still had some pain when she woke up in the morning, but this wore off once she was up and about.

I hypnotized her again and repeated the suggestions that I had given her on the previous occasion. I told her that, since she had mastered these techniques so quickly, she would find that she could control her pain, even if it came on at a time when it wasn't possible for her to lie down and practice her progressive relaxation. She would, in future, be able to relax her muscles and reduce the pain just by visualizing the golden light flowing down her back. I told her that from now on she would be able to control her back muscles as well as she could control her hand muscles and her face muscles. She could control her hands perfectly for writing, sewing and so on, and her face for eating and speaking. The back muscles were no different, so there was no reason why she shouldn't be able to control them just as well.

Donna's third appointment was a month later. She told me, with delight, that she had had nothing more than one episode of mild backache after doing some heavy housework. She knew now that she would not finish up in a wheelchair and this, in itself, had relieved a considerable amount of stress. She also noticed that she was feeling very much more relaxed in herself and that she was coping considerably better with situations which, previously, would have made her nervous and panicky.

I suggested that, if she had any more twinges, she might return to see the osteopath since, now the spasm had been dealt with, he should be able to restore her back to a state in which she would be totally free of pain.

A year later, Donna's husband 'phoned me to say that she had remained pain free since last seeing me and had just given birth to a baby girl.

DEBBIE

Debbie was 31 years old and happily married with three children aged ten, seven and four. She initially came to see me because she wanted some help in her attempt to lose weight. I gave her suggestions that she would not become hungry between meals and that she would be able to resist eating sweet foods and fatty foods. I told her that the foods which were allowed on her diet would start to taste so good that she wouldn't want to eat anything else. While she was still in trance, I asked her to project herself forward to the time when she would have lost the weight and to see herself looking in a mirror, admiring her new figure.

Because she was very keen to slim, the suggestions were rapidly effective and Debbie found that she was able to keep to the diet that she had set herself without any desire to break it. She got down to her target weight without difficulty and then returned to see me on another matter. Having responded so well to hypnosis herself, she wanted to know whether I could treat her seven year old son, who suffered badly from asthma. I explained to her that, with children that young, a lot depended on their ability to concentrate but, although one could never guarantee results, it was possible that hypnotherapy might help.

Because sometimes a parent can become so anxious about a child's asthma that this in itself can make the child worse, I asked Debbie about her reactions to the attacks. But she was a sensible woman and she said that she took the attacks in her stride, administering the medication prescribed by the doctor and calling him if the attack seemed to be getting bad. "It's upsetting to see Will like that but I try to reassure him," she said. "Anyway, I have great faith in our doctor, so that stops me from panicking."

I asked her about Will's general health and she told me that he was a fairly sturdy little boy "which is amazing really in view of the asthma and the fact that he had a difficult start to life". On questioning, it turned out that Will had been born prematurely and had spent the first four weeks of his life in an incubator. Debbie had not even been able to hold him until he was a few days old. From the first, he was fed with her milk, but she had needed to express it as he was too small to suck. And once she was able to start breast-feeding him, it was a while before he was able to take enough from her.

Although Will was never in danger, his parents were both very worried about him and Debbie thought that they had never quite lost this anxiety. Despite the fact that she tried to be sensible about his asthma, she and her husband were both inclined to fuss more over Will than over either of their other two children.

It was starting to sound as though Debbie and Will hadn't had a chance to bond at birth. Outwardly, it didn't seem to have affected the relationship between them but, from what she had said, it seemed very likely that Debbie and her husband, quite unconsciously, treated Will in a different way from his brother and sister.

As described in the section on asthma in chapter seven, regression to the time of Will's birth, with a 're-telling' of the story, could subtly adjust Debbie's attitude to him, both with regard to bonding and to her anxiety. When I explained the technique, she was keen to try it. Her doctor had no objection, so she made an appointment to start the treatment.

At the next session, I put Debbie into a hypnotic trance and used a few techniques to get her as deep as possible. The first part of the therapy was aimed at making her subconscious mind accept the suggestion that Will was not born at 34 weeks, but at 38 weeks—in other words, only two weeks early. I asked her to remember back to the day of her last appointment at the ante-natal clinic before Will was born.

"Picture yourself going in and giving your name to the receptionist at the desk. I expect you know her quite well by now, don't you?"
"Yes, it seems as though we're old friends."
"She's crossing you off her list and she's saying that this may be your last appointment before the baby's born. A lot of the ladies deliver a week or two early so, as you're now at 38 weeks, it could be any time now."

After a slight pause, I continued "Now go slightly further forward in time until you're in the cubicle, waiting to see the doctor. Are you lying on the couch?"
"Yes."
"What color gown are you wearing?"
"Blue." (Asking questions about details such as color can help the visualization to become clearer.)
"And now the doctor's coming in. What's his name?"
"Mr. Davidson."

"He's asking how you are. What are you telling him?"

"I feel fine."

"Good. Now he's going to have a feel of your tummy. He says the baby is a good size and is the right way up. He thinks it could be due any time. He's very pleased with you. Everything's going very well. He tells you to get dressed and says that he will see you again next week if you haven't yet had the baby. Otherwise, he'll see you on the ward."

I then asked Debbie to visualize further scenes in which hospital staff and friends commented on the fact that the baby must be almost due and that she would be going into hospital very soon. Having established that Will's birth, when it occurred, was not going to be premature, because she was 38 weeks pregnant, I took Debbie forward in time to when her labor pains began.

I asked her how she was feeling as she realized that she was going into labor and she said "Excited". This was a good indication that she had accepted the suggestion that Will would not be premature. If she had been anxious at going into premature labor, she would have been more likely to say 'nervous' or 'worried', rather than 'excited'. I asked her to relive the journey to the hospital, describing it as she went, and then to picture herself being admitted into the labor ward.

After this, I took her forward in time again, to a point just a few minutes before Will's birth. I asked her to describe the midwives who were looking after her and gave her suggestions such as "They're so kind. They make you feel so confident and happy." I told her to picture her husband by her side, holding her hand. (Because, in real life, this had been a premature birth, her husband hadn't been allowed to stay with her in case any emergency procedures were necessary.) Finally she described Will being born, with a minimum of pain, and how he started to cry straight away.

"And now the midwife has picked him up and wrapped him in a towel and is handing him to you. Take him and hold him. He's a lovely boy, fit and healthy. And you're so happy. Your husband's there too, and he's just as happy as you are."

In this way, Debbie was given an alternative story which her subconscious mind could use to replace the unhappy memories of the actual birth. Before waking her up, I told her that, while she would remember the birth as it actually happened, she would behave as though it had been the way she had just pictured it and she would no longer be affected by any problems that occurred at the time. When I brought her out of the trance, Debbie was smiling and happy.

Some weeks later, she 'phoned me to say that, although it was November, Will's asthma had been much less troublesome than usual. They had just been to the asthma clinic at the local hospital and the doctor had been so pleased with Will that he had reduced some of his medication.

I heard nothing more but, two years later, a chance meeting with Debbie in the street brought the story up to date. Will, she said, was now very well. He was doing well at school and was taking part in sports. His asthma attacks occurred only very rarely now and he no longer had to take medication all the time. The improvement, she said, dated from the 'bonding' session of hypnotherapy. Of course, some children do grow out of asthma and so hypnotherapy can't claim all the credit. However, Debbie's next remark was very interesting. She said "And since I had that hypnotherapy, Will and I have become so much closer—I've got a really wonderful relationship now with all my children".

ABIGAIL

The first hypnotherapy that Abigail had was as an emergency. She was a talented 17 year old dancer who was a full-time student at a ballet school and was hoping to dance professionally. Her school was putting on an evening of ballet excerpts and she had some important solos. However, at lunchtime on the day of the show, she started to develop a migraine. She had been suffering from migraines since the age of 14 and, recently, they had been getting more frequent. This was the second attack that she had had within four weeks. She had noticed that they were more likely to happen when she was nervous or under stress and she put the increased frequency down to the fact that she was studying for her A-level exams as well as working hard towards a dancing career.

Abigail was sent home from school to rest but by five o'clock she was no better. Her mother thought that she would have to ring the school to tell them to put on an understudy but decided, first of all, to speak to her family doctor to ask if there was anything he could prescribe that might help. The doctor suggested that she contact me and ask if I would do a home visit.

And so, at six o'clock, an hour and a half before the curtain was due to go up, Abigail had her first session of hypnosis. She was complaining of a severe throbbing pain in the right side of her head. The light hurt her eyes and she was lying in a darkened room. Any movement or touch made her headache worse, so she lay very still, with her eyes shut. She had vomited twice.

I explained to her that if she followed the instructions that I gave her, there was a good chance that her headache would be relieved. An incentive such as this often helps to get patients into hypnosis if they are in pain. She went into a trance easily and I then asked her to lay her hand against the part of her head where the pain was most severe. She did so, gingerly. I asked her to feel the warmth from her hand flowing into her head and soothing away and replacing the pain.

After about five minutes, during which I repeated the suggestion several times, she started to smile and said "It's going". After another few minutes, she said "It's gone". I told her that the headache would not return that evening, and then woke her up. Once awake, she was free of pain, but feeling rather weak. However, once she had had something to eat and drink, she felt well enough to go back to school and take part in the show.

As Abigail wanted to be a professional dancer, it was important that she should not be plagued by migraine every time she had an important role. She decided, therefore, to have some more hypnotherapy to try to get rid of the migraine for good.

Having experienced rapid pain relief in the first session, she was very receptive to the idea that hypnosis was going to work, and she went easily into a moderately deep trance. I taught her self-hypnosis and the 'clenched fist' technique described in the section on migraine in chapter seven. I advised her to practice self-hypnosis regularly.

Two weeks later, she returned for her next appointment and told me that, a few days earlier, she had been sitting watching television when she saw spots in front of her eyes and her vision became distorted—sure signs, for her, that a migraine was coming on. She immediately used the 'clenched fist' technique. Within a few minutes she was free of symptoms and no headache developed.

I saw Abigail once more, a month later, when she told me that she had had no further symptoms despite the fact that she was working very hard at the moment. Since she was still practicing self-hypnosis every day, she was confident that, if a migraine did start, she could control it without difficulty.

TOBY

When I was working as a family doctor, this 14 year old boy was brought in one morning by his mother. He had developed a large and painful abscess on his shoulder and his mother had decided that medical treatment was now necessary. The boy looked glum and said that he had "not wanted to bother the doctor" and that he was sure it would get better by itself.

On examination, however, the abscess was a large one and in obvious need of being opened and drained. When I told Toby this, he went very pale and it became clear that his reason for 'not wanting to bother me' had nothing to do with the conviction that the abscess would heal itself, but was solely due to the fact that he would rather have the abscess than the treatment.

I explained to Toby that, once the abscess had been incised, he would feel a lot better and that I would do it under local anesthetic, so that he wouldn't feel anything. But this was of little comfort to him since he was as scared of needles as he was of the incision and, in any case, he wasn't at all sure that the anesthetic would work. By this time, he was near to tears.

At this point, I told Toby that it was possible for me to teach him how to go into a nice dreamy state in which he would hardly be aware of what was going on. Knowing that his mother wouldn't allow him to leave the surgery until the abscess had been treated, he agreed to this. So I asked him to lie down on the couch and I put him into hypnosis.

Once he was in a trance, I asked him to imagine that he was sitting in front of the television at home, watching his favourite program. I gave him a moment and then asked if he could see it.

"Yes," he replied. "It's just starting".
"Can you see the titles coming up on the screen and hear the signature tune?"

"Yes."

"Keep watching and listening and, as you do, the picture and the sound will become clearer and clearer, until they will both be as clear as if you were watching the program at home. And you will find the program so interesting and so enjoyable that you won't pay any attention at all to what I'm doing. Even if you feel some discomfort, it won't worry you—you will be so interested in what's happening on the television that nothing will distract you from it until I tell you that it's time to wake up."

And this is exactly what happened. Toby lay there, smiling to himself as he ran an edition of his favourite program through his mind. And I injected local anesthetic and incised and drained the abscess without him flinching once. When I'd finished dressing the wound, I told Toby that the program was finishing and that the closing credits were coming up. Then I brought him out of trance and asked how the program had been and how he felt. He answered "Great!" to both questions.

This 'television' technique is one which is popular with dentists who treat children, and it is particularly useful when treatment is necessary which will entail the child either being in the chair for a long period of time or returning on several occasions. When a number of appointments are necessary, the child may be asked to decide in advance which program to watch on the next visit and, as a result, may almost look forward to the trips to the dentist.

MARGARET

Margaret was a highly intelligent, well-educated young woman of 24 who worked as a translator for a large publishing house. While in her last year at university, she had met an American post-graduate student to whom she had been very attracted. They had been 'an item' for a year and, when he returned to the United States, they had emailed and 'phoned each other regularly.

Four months before Margaret came for hypnotherapy, her boyfriend returned to England for an extended holiday before taking up a post at a British university. Towards the end of this holiday, he asked her to marry him and she said yes. Now he wanted her to go to America to meet his family, but she was terrified of flying. Her fiancé had already returned home and she would have to travel alone, which made the prospect even more alarming. Because she was under pressure at work, it wasn't possible for her to take more than a two week break, so she couldn't travel by sea. She knew she could force herself to book the flight and even to get to the airport, but she didn't know whether she could actually force herself to get on the plane—and if she couldn't, she would risk losing the man she loved.

Margaret had flown twice before. At the age of fourteen she had taken a plane home from Paris where she had been on holiday with some relatives. They were staying in France for another week but she had to return to England for the start of the school term. On the outward journey they had traveled by car and boat but, since she would now be traveling alone, her parents thought it was safer for her to fly.

She had not been nervous when she got on the plane but, unfortunately, the weather was bad and the flight was a very bumpy one. Even more unfortunately, she was sitting next to a woman who regaled her with information about planes crashing in storms, and when she got off at the other end to be met by her parents, she was trembling and tearful.

After that, she was able to avoid flying for seven years but then had to fly to Edinburgh where her mother, who had been visiting a friend, had suddenly become seriously ill. On this occasion, Margaret traveled with her father and, in view of her anxiety about her mother and her fear of flying, her doctor gave her some tranquilizers to take for the journey. These had suppressed her panic to some extent but, once her mother had recovered and Margaret returned home, she was thankful to be able to do so on the train.

Although taking tranquilizers had helped to control Margaret's anxiety when she had to fly to Edinburgh, she remembered that she had felt very drowsy and "like a zombie" on her arrival. As the flight to the United States was so much longer than that to Edinburgh, she was afraid that, if she were to take tranquilizers, she would need a larger dose and that, by the time she arrived, she would be in no fit state to meet her future in-laws. She went to see her doctor and explained her dilemma, and he suggested that she try hypnotherapy.

When she came for her first session, Margaret had managed to book her ticket for a flight in three weeks' time. She had explained the delay to her fiancé by saying that she had some urgent work to complete before she could take any holiday. But she was afraid that, if she delayed any longer, he would think that she was having second thoughts about marrying him.

Once she was in a hypnotic trance, I told Margaret that, in future, she would not have any difficulty in relaxing and staying calm, whatever the circumstances. (In fact, she was normally a very relaxed person and the only thing that made her panic was the thought of flying.) I used a couple of techniques to develop her sense of relaxation and well-being and then asked her to visualize herself packing her suitcase, ready for her trip to the States. As she did so, I gave her suggestions that not only was she remaining relaxed but she was getting quite excited at the thought of seeing her fiancé again and of meeting his family.

Then I asked her to change the scene to the airport. I told her that it is natural, if we are under stress or having to do something out of the ordinary, for the body to release adrenaline into the system. When we are anxious or feel threatened, this can be an unpleasant sensation and can intensify the anxiety but, when we are happy, it can produce a feeling of excitement. In this case, because she was happy and looking forward to seeing her fiancé again, her mind would interpret the sensation as being one of excitement and it would add to her happiness.

I then continued to take her through the visualization of going through the formalities at the airport. Each time she started to feel nervous or apprehensive, she 'froze' the scene until the sensation turned into one of excitement. Finally, she was able to picture herself getting onto the plane and starting the flight. I asked her to feel herself becoming very relaxed and, when asked, she said that she felt very calm and relaxed and comfortable.

After this, I taught her self-hypnosis and told her that, once on the plane, she would be able to put herself into a trance and remain comfortably relaxed throughout the journey, which would seem to pass very quickly. She would be aware of any announcements being made, so she would know when to wake up at the end of the flight and also when meals were being served. If she woke up to eat or if she needed to wake herself up to go to the toilet, she would remain quite calm and would be able to go back into hypnosis as soon as she wanted to.

Of course, I included the usual self-hypnosis precautions— "If anything should happen that needs your immediate attention, you will wake up immediately and, while remaining calm, will be fully alert to deal with it"—making sure that I said it in a way that didn't suggest that there *would* be an emergency on the plane!

Margaret had two more sessions of hypnosis before her trip. At each, I repeated all the suggestions and techniques that I had used on the first occasion. She practiced her self-hypnosis diligently and, by the end of her third appointment, was feeling fairly confident about the flight.

204

When the time came for her journey, the flight was uneventful and Margaret accomplished it with a minimum of anxiety. She was able to wake up to have something to eat but spent the rest of the time in hypnosis and found that the journey passed quickly. She had a wonderful time in the States and coped well with the flight home. And, three months later, she and her fiancé were married—and flew to Bermuda for their honeymoon.

MALLORY

Although there are certain areas of medicine in which hypnosis can't be of use, the fact that it can be combined with other therapeutic techniques makes it very valuable in the treatment of a great variety of complaints. Not only can it be used together with many forms of orthodox medicine, but it can also supplement other complementary therapies. Any therapy that uses visualization can be combined with hypnosis to very good effect.

Visualization can be a very powerful technique and its use in the treatment of cancer was pioneered in the United States by Carl Simonton and Stephanie Matthews-Simonton (authors, with James L. Creighton, of *Getting Well Again*, Bantam, 1986). Healing (sometimes called spiritual healing, psychic healing or hand healing) can also make use of visualizations through which patients can use the power of their own minds to help heal their bodies.

I treated Mallory with a combination of hypnosis and a healing visualization. When I was working in general practice, she came in one day, having just fallen over in the street, cutting her leg quite badly. I cleaned and stitched the cut and, while I was doing so, Mallory mentioned that she was "always doing things like this". She went on to tell me that she was very accident prone. But many of the accidents, it seemed, were not of her own making. Hardly a day went by without something happening to her and she was getting heartily fed up with it. The day before she fell over in the street, someone had run into the back of her car when she had stopped at traffic lights. Two days before that, when changing the bed linen, one of the pillows had suddenly given way and filled the room with feathers. And to make matters worse, when she got out the vacuum cleaner to clear up the mess, she found that it wasn't working.

Now a healer might say that the reason that Mallory was accident prone was because she was surrounded by negative energies. The energy, or life force, that runs through the body has to flow in an ordered manner; if it is disrupted it can cause disease or abnormal mental states or, as in this case, can disturb the patient's environment. (The phenomenon of the poltergeist, in which inanimate objects are hurled across the room and doors open and shut of their own accord, is often associated with the presence in the household of a disturbed teenager.)

Knowing something about healing techniques, I decided to use a healing visualization and to combine this with hypnosis which would not only make the visualization easier for her but would also allow me to give her some ego-strengthening and teach her to relax. I hoped that, using this combination, something might help!

206

The method I used was based on a technique described in *The Psychic Healing Book* by Amy Wallace and Bill Henkin (North Atlantic Books, 2004). Once Mallory was in hypnosis and I had given her some basic suggestions regarding relaxation and ego-strengthening, I asked her to focus on a point just in front of the base of her spine. When she indicated that she had done so (by raising a finger), I asked her to imagine that, lying there, was a cord which had been rolled up into a ball. Again, she indicated that she could see the cord. I asked her to picture it unrolling and running down through the chair on which she was sitting, into the ground and right down to the centre of the earth, where it would anchor itself.

I told Mallory that this cord could be used for 'waste disposal', to get rid of all the disturbed energies that she was sure she was surrounded by. I asked her to imagine that she was sweeping round her body with her hands, scooping up any 'muck' that surrounded her and transferring it to the top of the cord. It would then flow down the cord, just like garbage going down a waste disposal unit and, when it got to the centre of the earth, it would disperse so that it could harm no one.

When she had been all round her body with her imaginary hands, and had cleared away as much as she could, I asked Mallory to draw up through the cord a clear, fresh, bubbling energy and use it to wash through and round her body to flush any remaining garbage down the cord. I suggested she repeat this step as many times as she needed to, flushing the used energy down the cord each time, until she felt clean and fresh. And then I asked her to draw up a final lot of energy which she could keep in her body. After this, I taught her self-hypnosis and suggested that she use the cord visualization every time she hypnotized herself, in order to rid herself of any anxieties or tensions that she had picked up during the day.

When Mallory returned two weeks later for her follow-up appointment, she reported that she had had only one minor accident since I had seen her last. She had been practicing her self-hypnosis every day and was feeling confident that she had freed herself from the accident prone tendency. I suggested she continue to practice the technique and to return if the problem showed any sign of coming back. She came back to the medical centre six months later—but, on this occasion, it was because she had a bad cough. The accident prone tendency was a thing of the past.

KATE

Kate was a 35 year old widow who worked as a buyer in a store and had two daughters aged 14 and 12. Her husband had died from leukemia two years earlier after several months of illness, much of which was spent in hospital. About a year after his death, Kate had experienced an attack of depression which quickly resolved with a course of antidepressant tablets.

She had come for hypnosis because she was a heavy smoker. She had started when she was in her late teens and, although she had sometimes managed to give up for a few weeks, she had always started again. I gave her the standard 'stop-smoking' treatment, with suggestions on how easy it was going to be to give up, and I taught her how to hypnotize herself. Self-hypnosis can induce depression in susceptible

208

patients but, in this case, it seemed that her one attack of depression had been a reaction to her husband's death and was unlikely to recur. However, as a precaution, after I had brought her out of the trance, I warned her that if she started to feel even the slightest bit depressed she should stop her practice immediately.

Two weeks later, Kate returned. Not only was she still smoking, but she had become very depressed. When she had had the first attack of depression, she had accepted it as being 'one of those things', but its sudden recurrence after two sessions of self-hypnosis, together with my warning, had started her wondering why she should be susceptible to depression, as she now appeared to be. As a result, she had come to some surprising conclusions. She had not, she said, been very happy with her life since her husband's death but she had become so used to bottling up her feelings "for the sake of the girls" that she was fooling even herself. She missed her husband enormously but had "shut the emotions away and just got on with things".

I asked her if she had really mourned her husband. She admitted that she had shed very few tears. All through his illness she had tried to keep cheerful for him, and when he was gone she had tried to keep cheerful for the girls, who were distraught at losing their father. I suggested that what she really needed was to allow herself to grieve. Kate agreed to talk to her daughters about the fact that she sometimes felt very lonely and needed to cry.

I put her into hypnosis and gave her suggestions that she would allow herself to weep and to mourn. But, by doing so, she would begin to feel great relief, as though a weight was lifting from her shoulders. Gradually all the pain and sadness would disappear and she would be left with happy memories of her husband. The grief of losing him would be replaced by thankfulness that she had known him and loved him and had been loved by him, and joy that he had given her two wonderful daughters.

I asked Kate to get in touch again if she needed further help, but I didn't give her another appointment. Six months later, I received a letter from her in which she said that she had allowed herself to mourn and to grieve deeply, helped and supported by her daughters and by a close friend at work. She had now cast off the depression and could think of her husband with smiles rather than tears. She was a great deal happier than she had been for several years and, during the last three weeks, had not smoked a single cigarette.

CHARLIE

Like Kate, Charlie came for hypnotherapy to help him stop smoking. He was a very good subject and it seemed that he would have little difficulty in giving up, since he had the motivation to do so.

At his second appointment, he mentioned that he was due to go into hospital as a day patient in order to have some little fatty nodules removed from under his eyes. He asked whether he might put himself into hypnosis for the duration of the operation, which was to be done under local anaesthetic. This seemed a very sensible idea — not only would he be very relaxed, but hypnosis has the effect of controlling bleeding and so might help to reduce the bruising that was likely to occur afterwards. (The area around the eyes is very sensitive and the surgeon had warned Charlie that he might have considerable bruising for a week or so after the operation.)

When he arrived at the hospital for his operation, Charlie spoke to the surgeon and, finding that he had no objection, put himself into trance while the fatty lumps were removed. A week later, he returned to see me for another session of hypnotherapy, by which time he had stopped smoking. I asked how the operation had gone and he told me that not only had he remained perfectly relaxed and comfortable throughout but, much to the surgeon's surprise, he had developed no bruising whatsoever.

DANNY

Danny was a successful businessman who had an impacted wisdom tooth. He was frequently in pain because he developed recurrent abscesses in his gums which needed to be treated with antibiotics. His dentist told him that he would have to have the tooth removed. It was the only way to prevent the abscesses from occurring. Danny accepted this — he wanted to be free of pain. He just couldn't bring himself to make the appointment at the hospital.

The underlying problem was Danny's fear of blood. He was afraid that, if he saw any blood or tasted it in his mouth, he would pass out and make a fool of himself. He was as frightened of 'weakness', of feeling faint and of not being in control as he was of blood. Interestingly, the thought of having an injection of local anesthetic in his mouth didn't worry him at all.

One of the first things that I noticed about Danny was that he was very fidgety. I mentioned this and he said that he had never been able to relax fully. I suggested that, before we started doing anything about his wisdom tooth problem, we spend a session using hypnosis to help him relax. Somewhat to my surprise, he proved to be an excellent subject and went into trance quickly and easily. I taught him self-hypnosis and gave various ego-strengthening suggestions.

When Danny came for his next appointment, he said that he had practiced self-hypnosis regularly but was concerned that his trance was very light. We therefore used the session to repeat what we had done before, going over the self-hypnosis instructions again and giving him suggestions that he would be able to put himself into trance very successfully.

Two weeks later, he reported that he was finding it much easier to induce self-hypnosis and was ready to tackle the problem of the wisdom tooth. But, when I tried to put him into hypnosis, he seemed to be fighting it. I asked him what was happening and he said that, although he could now relax much better, he didn't actually like relaxing because he felt that he wasn't in control. I suggested, therefore, that he put himself into hypnosis—and he achieved this very easily. He allowed me to use some deepening techniques and, once he was in a medium depth trance, I asked him to do a visualization. He knew the hospital where he was due to go for the operation and so was able to picture it easily. I suggested that he picture himself in the car, with his wife, traveling to the hospital. Then I asked him to jump forward in time and see himself arriving and parking the car. After this, he pictured himself going into the hospital, reporting to reception and being sent to the dental department waiting room. He saw himself sitting down in a chair, waiting to be called in.

All the time that Danny was doing the visualization, I was giving him suggestions that he was feeling calm, confident and relaxed. After a few moments in the waiting room, I asked him to see himself being called in to see the surgeon and sitting in the dental chair. Finally, I suggested he fast-forward the picture and see himself getting up out of the chair, having had the tooth removed, and walking back into the waiting room with a big smile on his face. I also suggested that he would be able to put himself into hypnosis in the dental chair, with the surgeon's approval, and would wake up when the surgeon put his hand on Danny's shoulder and said his name. When I woke him up, he said he was feeling much more confident.

He contacted me ten days later to say that he had had the tooth removed and, although he had felt slightly nervous, he had coped very well. In fact, the surgeon had said that he was the best patient he'd had all week!

CHAPTER NINE: HAVING THERAPY

WHEN, AND FOR WHOM, IS HYPNOTHERAPY SUITABLE?

In some respects, hypnotherapy has more in common with orthodox medicine than with complementary therapies. In therapies such as homeopathy, acupuncture and radionics, the aim of treatment is to return the patient to as near normal a state as possible. But in orthodox medicine, although some forms of treatment may cure the patient, some may only control the condition (for example, drugs given to treat high blood pressure or arthritis) and some may just alleviate the symptoms (such as aspirin taken for pain).

Similarly, there are some conditions that hypnosis can cure (such as phobias and chronic anxiety, where the patient can be helped to recognize and conquer the cause) but it may be able only to control others (for example, cases of migraine or asthma where the patient needs to use a certain technique every time an attack begins in order to stop it from developing). And in some cases hypnosis will only alleviate the symptoms—as in the case of chronic pain. But when the patient has tried other available treatments without success, even a therapy that will only control the condition or alleviate the symptoms will be welcome.

So when should you consider having hypnotherapy and when should you try another complementary therapy? Should hypnosis always be a last resort? The answer to this second question is definitely no. Any patient whose condition is directly related to stress or anxiety might be well advised to try hypnotherapy first. And for a patient who suffers from a physical condition such as asthma, which is aggravated by anxiety or stress, hypnosis can be very successfully combined with orthodox treatment.

However, for the treatment of pain, hypnotherapy should probably come last on the list, simply because all it will do is cover up the symptoms. But, that said, there can be cases, such as that of the woman who suffered from back pain (described in chapter eight), in which anxiety and tension play such a large part in the production of the pain that hypnotherapy may relieve it simply by teaching the patient how to relax. Normally, for back problems, osteopathy or chiropractic would probably be the treatment of first choice, but severe muscle spasm may prevent the patient from responding.

The cases in which hypnotherapy excels are those in which the patient is suffering from anxiety and does not wish to take tranquilizers. Since many doctors are becoming increasingly reluctant to prescribe tranquilizers, they are often happy to refer patients for other, non-addictive forms of treatment.

Sometimes people are put off the idea of hypnotherapy because they have tried listening to self-hypnosis CDs or mp3s and have found them unhelpful. However, it's important to recognize that, while such recordings may be very beneficial to some people, their use is limited. They may, certainly, induce a light hypnotic trance, and some people who simply need to relax or who are trying to give up smoking may find that they are perfectly adequate for their purposes.

But a trance that you induce yourself is unlikely to be as deep as a trance induced by a therapist. It does seem that better results are to be achieved from a session with a therapist than from a session, or sessions, with an iPod or CD player. In addition, the session that you have with a hypnotherapist will be tailor-made to your own personal problems. In the case of smokers, for example, specific suggestions can be given to help them to deal with the times when they find it most difficult to refrain from lighting up.

If someone is suffering from a particular mental or physical condition, specific and appropriate suggestions are even more important. People who suspect that they are depressed should exercise caution in using self-hypnosis recordings and, if they do and start to feel more depressed after listening to one, they should stop using it immediately.

If you have decided that you might benefit from hypnotherapy, you then need to look for a qualified therapist. This means someone who has been properly trained and is registered with a recognized hypnotherapy organisation.

WHAT WILL HAPPEN AND HOW MUCH WILL IT COST?

The cost of hypnotherapy will vary from country to country and from therapist to therapist. Many practitioners offer reduced rates to patients who can't afford the full fees so, if this applies to you, enquire about it when you 'phone or email to make an appointment.

The session itself also varies according to the individual therapist and, of course, the condition that is being treated. However, as a general rule, sessions last between one and two hours. At the first session, the therapist will take a full history and may enquire into your family background and childhood as well as noting the details of the present problem.

Some practitioners don't give any treatment in the first session but simply explain to patients the lines upon which they intend to treat them and then answer any questions they might have. This is often the course taken with children for whom it is very important to engender a sense of trust before the treatment begins.

If hypnosis is induced in the first session, it is usually quite short, since time has been spent on taking the history and discussing the proposed treatment. The patient may be given a few suggestions concerning relaxation and ego-strengthening and may be taught self-hypnosis.

The length of treatment and frequency of sessions depend very much on the individual patient and the complaint being treated. Patients may be seen weekly or fortnightly to begin with and then, as their condition starts to improve, less often. Some may need to continue treatment for many months, particularly those who are suffering from severe and chronic phobias. Others, such as those who wish to give up smoking, may need only two or three sessions.

Whatever the condition being treated, one would normally expect some improvement, even if only slight, within four or five sessions. No change in the condition after five sessions suggests that perhaps the patient should try a different therapy.

There are a few conditions that hypnosis may make worse, including some forms of depression and schizophrenia. If you see a properly qualified therapist (in other words, one who has a background in medicine or psychotherapy) you will be advised, before you start, whether hypnosis is right for you.

It is important to remember that hypnotherapy is not a cure-all and has definite limitations. However, alone or combined with other therapies, it may produce a dramatic improvement in a patient's condition, especially when that condition is aggravated by stress.

FINDING A THERAPIST

If you want to see a medical hypnotherapist, you may need to get a referral letter from your own doctor, depending on the country you live in. But, no matter where you live, it is essential that the therapist you choose has had proper training and has professional indemnity insurance. A therapist who is a member of a recognized professional body will have to abide by the code of conduct that organization lays down, and this is an additional safety factor.

Many dentists use hypnosis for patients with dental phobias and to relieve pain during dental treatment. Some of these may have done additional training so that they can offer additional hypnotherapeutic treatment—for example to help patients to stop smoking—but others will use it only for dentistry.

Unfortunately, hypnotherapy is not as well regulated as some other therapies and there are many different societies and organizations which register practitioners, so it is sometimes hard to know quite how thorough a training the therapist has had. If in doubt, it is always best to choose someone who has a qualification in medicine or psychotherapy in addition to hypnosis. Professor Martin Orne (see chapter two) has been quoted as saying "If a person is not professionally qualified to treat something without hypnosis, then they're not qualified to treat something with hypnosis, either. First you look for that professional certificate on the wall—physician, dentist, clinical psychologist, or whatever. Then you look for the certificate of hypnosis."

The following organizations hold registers of physicians, dentists, psychologists and psychotherapists who are also hypnotherapists. Where the register is available online, I have given a direct link to it. Where there is a 'phone number, I have given that too.

Australia
ASH: Australian Society of Hypnosis
http://www.hypnosisaustralia.org.au/seekingtreatment/referral-list/

This link can be used to find a therapist in New South Wales, South Australia or Victoria.

For therapists in other parts of the country, email:
for Tasmania: ashltd@optusnet.com.au
for Queensland: jamesauld@bigpond.com
for Western Australia: brianallenassoc@yahoo.com.au
(or phone +61 8 9322 4219).
Main office: tel: +61 2 9747 4691

Austria
ÖGATAP: Austrian Society for Applied Depth Psychology and General Psychotherapy
http://www.oegatap.at/therapeutensuche
Tel: 01523 38 39 (Mon.-Thurs. 10.00-13.00)

MEGA: Milton Erickson Society for Clinical Hypnosis and Brief Therapy, Austria
http://www.hypno-mega.at/hypnotherapeuten-absolventenliste.html
Tel: +43 (0) 660 577 90 09

Belgium
VHYP: Vlaams Wetenschappelijke Hypnose Vereniging (Flemish Society of Scientific Hypnosis)
http://www.vhyp.be/hypnotherapeuten-in-uw-regio

Canada
SQH: Société Québécoise d'Hypnose
http://sqh.info/liste-membres/
Tel: 514-990-1205

Denmark
DSCH: Danish Society of Clinical Hypnosis
http://hypnoseselskabet.dk/behandler-kort/

Finland
NVVH: Tieteellinen Hypnoosi ry, Vetenskaplig Hypnos rf (Finland Society for Scientific Hypnosis)
http://www.hypnoosi.net/paakaupunki.html

France

AFHYP: Association Française d'Hypnose
http://www.afhyp.fr/annuaire_v67.php

AFEHM: Association Française pour l'Etude de l'Hypnose Médicale
http://www.hypnosemedicale.com/trouver+un+therapeute/
(Click on appropriate area of map)
Tel: +33 (0) 1 42 56 65 65

Emergences: Institut de Formation et de Recherche en Hypnose et Communication Thérapeutique
http://www.hypnoses.com/annuaire-hypnose/
Tel: +33 (0) 9 62 16 34 17

IMHETO: Institut Milton H. Erickson de Toulouse
http://www.atnh.net/ATNHdev/annuaire/
Tel: +33 (0) 5 34 42 18 75

Institut Milton H. Erickson de Biarritz-Pays Basque
http://hypnosium.com/annuaire-des-praticiens/
Tel: +33 (0) 6 03 85 60 26

Institut Milton H. Erickson de Méditerranée — ToulonMarseille
http://hypnose-medicale.com/wp-content/themes/twentytwelve/
img/2015-liste-hypnotherapeutes.pdf
Tel: +33 (0) 4 94 18 97 22

SFH — Société Française d'Hypnose
http://www.hypnose-sfh.com/annuaire-adherer/
Tel: +33 (0) 1 48 04 92 96

Germany
DGHH: German Society of Hypnosis and Hypnotherapy
http://www.hypnose-dgh.de/therapeutenliste.html

DGZH: German Society of Dental Hypnosis
http://www.rent-a-brain.de/dgzh/aerzteliste.php?public=1&order=addnames.
add_name2&listenart=Hypnosezahnaerzte&ordertext=Nachname
Tel: 0711-23 60618 Mon to Fri: 9:00 — 13:00;
Mon to Thurs 14:00 — 17:00

DGAHAT
Deutsche Gesellschaft fur Arztliche Hypnose und Autogenes Training
http://www.dgaehat.de/ueber-uns/therapeuten/
Email: info@dgaehat.de

Hungary
MHE: Magyar Hipnozis Egyesulet
http://www.hipnozis-mhe.hu/index.php?option=com_
content&view=article&id=9&Itemid=5

Iceland
IcSH: The Icelandic Society of Hypnosis
http://www.dfi.is/thjonusta/

India
ISCEH: Indian Society of Clinical and Experimental Hypnosis
http://hypnosissocietyindia.org/membership.htm (List of
members with links to individual websites)

Israel
IsSH: Israel Society of Hypnosis
http://www.hebpsy.net/pl.asp?method=45&prof=1

Italy
CIICS: Italian Centre for Clinical and Experimental Hypnosis
Has a register of members but not online
Tel. 011 74.99.601

SII: Italian Society of Hypnosis
http://www.societaipnosi.it/index.php?option=com_assoweb
&view=visualizzasoci&id_status_list=0&Itemid=117

for Sardinia   tel. 3389850550
for Tuscany-Umbria   tel. 3477698709
for Triveneto   tel. 045534271/3338364591

Luxembourg
IMHELUX: Institut Milton H. Erickson du Luxembourg
http://www.institutmiltonericksonluxembourg.com/liste-de-praticiens.html

Morocco
AMHYC: Association Marocaine d'Hypnose Clinique
http://www.amhyc.ma/?page=annuaire
Tel: 0522398722

Netherlands
NvvH: Netherlands Society of Hypnosis
Tel: 085-90 22 839

Norway
NSCEH: Norwegian Society of Clinical and Evidence-based Hypnosis
http://hypnoseforeningen.snappages.com/finn-behandler.htm

Poland
P-I-E: Polski Instytut Ericksonowski
Tel: (42) 688 48 60

South Africa
SASCH: South African Society of Clinical Hypnosis
http://www.sasch.co.za/find-a-therapist.html
Tel: 010 211 9024

Sweden
SSCH Swedish Society for Clinical Hypnosis
http://www.hypnosforeningen.se/behandlare.htm
Tel: 031-711 71 18

Switzerland

GHYPS: Gesellschaft fur klinische Hypnose Schweiz Société médicale (Society of Clinical Hypnosis Switzerland)
http://www.hypnos.ch/index.php
Tel: 031 911 47 10

SMSH: Swiss Medical Society of Hypnosis
http://www.smsh.ch/interessenten/therapeuten_plz.htm
Tel: 041 281 17 45

United Kingdom

BSCAH: British Society of Clinical and Academic Hypnosis
http://www.bscah.com/members/referral-list/
Tel: 07702 492867

BSMDH-S: British Society of Medical and Dental Hypnosis — Scotland
http://www.bsmdhscotland.com/find-a-therapist
Tel: 07981 333391

Counselling Directory
Hypnotherapists listed include members of BACP (British Association for Counselling and Psychotherapy) and UKCP (UK Council for Psychotherapy). Check the individual listing to ensure that the therapist is an accredited member of one of these organisations.
http://www.counselling-directory.org.uk/adv-search.html

USA

ASCH: American Society of Clinical Hypnosis
http://www.asch.net/Public/MemberReferralSearch.aspx
Tel: (630) 980-4740

SCEH: The Society for Clinical and Experimental Hypnosis
APA: The Society of Psychological Hypnosis

Members of both these organizations (as well as members of ASCH) can be found on the Societies of Hypnosis website:
https://www.societiesofhypnosis.com/disclaimer

INDEX

Printed in May 2023
by Rotomail Italia S.p.A., Vignate (MI) - Italy